# Essentials of To Medicine and Surgery

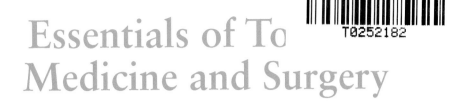

T0252182

**John Chitty**

*Anton Vets, Andover, Hampshire, UK*

**Aidan Raftery**

*Avian and Exotic Animal Clinic, Manchester, UK*

**WILEY** Blackwell

This edition first published 2013
© 2013 John Chitty and Aidan Raftery

*Registered Office*
John Wiley & Sons, Ltd, The Atrium, Southern Gate, Chichester, West Sussex, PO19 8SQ, UK

*Editorial Offices*
9600 Garsington Road, Oxford, OX4 2DQ, UK
The Atrium, Southern Gate, Chichester, West Sussex, PO19 8SQ, UK
350 Main Street, Malden, MA 02148-5020, USA

For details of our global editorial offices, for customer services and for information about
how to apply for permission to reuse the copyright material in this book please see our website at
www.wiley.com/wiley-blackwell

*Library of Congress Cataloging-in-Publication Data*

Chitty, John, MRCVS.
   Essentials of tortoise medicine and surgery / John Chitty, Aidan Raftery.
     p. ; cm.
   Includes bibliographical references and index.
   ISBN 978-1-4051-9544-7 (pbk. : alk. paper) – ISBN 978-1-118-65637-2 – ISBN 978-1-118-58399-9 (epdf) –
ISBN 978-1-118-58398-2 (epub) – ISBN 978-1-118-58396-8 (mobi)
   I. Raftery, Aidan.  II. Title.
   [DNLM:  1. Animal Diseases–therapy.  2. Turtles–physiology.  3. Animal Diseases–diagnosis.
4. Turtles–surgery.  SF 997.5.T87]
   SF459.T8
   639.3'924–dc23

                             2013010798

A catalogue record for this book is available from the British Library.

Wiley also publishes its books in a variety of electronic formats. Some content that appears in print may not be
available in electronic books.

Cover images: courtesy of John Chitty and Aidan Raftery
Cover design by Andy Meaden

Set in 10/12pt Sabon by SPi Publisher Services, Pondicherry, India

# Contents

# Preface

This book is designed to be a practical help for busy clinicians seeing Chelonia as part of their caseload.

It is not intended to be a complete textbook of tortoise diseases – for this, readers are referred to McArthur, Wilkinson and Meyer's *Medicine and Surgery of Tortoises and Turtles* (Blackwell Publishing, Oxford, 2004). More, it is intended to assist the clinician inexperienced with these species as a practical guide to assist in investigation of these occasionally seen species: hence its emphasis on the more common/likely diagnoses rather than completeness. It is based on our joint experiences in practising with these species over several decades. The species too are biased towards those more commonly seen in UK and US practices, rather than a complete overview of chelonid diseases.

To assist in this, the book may be considered in two parts – the first gives an overview of the basics of tortoise and semi-aquatic/aquatic freshwater turtle husbandry and keeping, as well as a guide to the general investigation and diagnostic techniques open to clinicians.

The second part is based on differential diagnosis and investigation by clinical signs. This does result in some repetition between sections, though we trust this will be balanced by an ease in following through a particular clinical sign! Disease syndromes and infectious agents are discussed within these sections, as patients tend to present with signs rather than diagnostic labels! A few exceptions are made for more complex syndromes that require more explanation or that are referenced from many different clinical signs; for example, hepatic lipidosis and follicular stasis.

In summary, we hope that this book will provide a useful guide and summary for the inexperienced and helping hand for those students, technicians/nurses and clinicians wishing to start advancing their knowledge of chelonian medicine. For more experienced clinicians and technicians working with these species, we hope that it will provide a useful aide memoire.

We would like to thank our colleagues and the owners of our patients for much assistance over many years. We would also like to thank the team at Wiley Blackwell for all their help and assistance during the long writing period. Most of all, we would like to thank our families for help, support and forbearance of long-term absenteeism!

John Chitty and Aidan Raftery

# Introduction

# 1 Biology

## 1.1 Species and Family Overview

This first section provides details on how to identify the different species described in this book.

Below is a brief description of the present-day families. The classification of species (and hence their scientific names) changes as we learn more about how closely they are related to other species. Most texts quickly become out of date as the taxonomists and systematists learn more about the relationship between and within different species. For an in-depth description with identification keys, the reader is directed to specialist publications such as Ernst and Barbour's *Turtles of the World* and Ferri's *Turtles and Tortoises*, which are good texts that provide more detailed information (see Figures 1.4.1 and 1.4.2 for scute nomenclature).

**Cheloniidae**   The six species of hard-shelled Sea turtles.

**Carettochelyidae**   This family has only one living species, the Pig-nosed turtle. The forelimbs are modified as flippers. It has a pig-like snout, and a smooth carapace from which scutes are absent.

**Dermochelyidae**   There is only one species in this family, the Leatherback sea turtle.

**Trionychidae**   There are approximately 22 species in this family of semi-aquatic turtles, which comprises the soft-shell turtles. The shell is reduced and incomplete. The carapace is leathery and pliable, particularly at the sides. They have elongated, soft, snorkel-like nostrils. Their necks are disproportionately long in comparison to their bodies.

**Kinosternidae**   Approximately 22 species are recognised in this family, which consists of the Mud turtles and the Musk turtles. Usually, one or two plastral hinges present.

*Essentials of Tortoise Medicine and Surgery*, First Edition. John Chitty and Aidan Raftery.
© 2013 John Chitty and Aidan Raftery. Published 2013 by John Wiley & Sons, Ltd.

They have less than 12 plastron scutes. Some degree of toe webbing is present. They are small- to medium-sized semi-aquatic turtles.

**Dermatemydidae**   There is one species, the Central American River turtle, which is almost totally aquatic. Inframarginal scutes are present.

**Platysternidae**   There is one species, the Big-headed turtle. The head is so big that it cannot be withdrawn into the shell. Inframarginal scutes are present.

**Chelydridae**   There are four living species, the Alligator snapping turtle and three species of Snapping turtles. These are very aggressive turtles, with powerful jaws. Inframarginal scutes are present. There is a long tail. The rough carapace is keeled and strongly serrated posteriorly. The plastron is reduced and hingeless.

**Testudinidae**   There are approximately 50 living species. This is the most common family presented for veterinary treatment in Europe. The hind limbs are columnar. Inframarginal scutes are absent. There are two phalangeal bones in the digits of the hind feet. There is no webbing of the toes. The genus *Kinixys* are the only tortoises with a hinge of the carapace. If a plastron hinge is present between the femoral and abdominal scutes, then the tortoise is in the genus *Testudo*, with the exception of *Testudo horsfieldi* (Horsfield's tortoise), which is recognisable by the horny claw on the end of its tail and by having only four claws on each forefoot. If the hinge is between the humeral and pectoral scutes, then this is *Pyxis arachnoides*, the Malagasy Spider tortoise. If the plastron is rigid with a very flat and flexible carapace, then this is *Malacochersus*, the Pancake tortoise. These are tortoises with paired gulars that project anteriorly beyond the carapace rim, especially in males and in the genus *Gopherus*, the Gopher tortoises. Where the supracaudal scute is undivided, then the tortoise is of the genus *Geochelone*.

### Guide to identification to the genera of the Testudinidae

**Kinixys**   This genus contains six species. They are the only tortoises with a movable hinge in the carapace. Three species are seen relatively commonly. In *Kinixys homeana* (Home's hinge-back tortoise), the posterior portion of the carapace is strongly inverted from the level of the anterior end of the fifth vertebral scute. The inversion of the carapace starts at the middle of the fifth vertebral scute in *K. erosa* (the Serrated hinge-back tortoise) and *K. belliana* (Bell's hinge-back tortoise). The posterior rim of the carapace of *K. erosa* is strongly serrated, while the same area of *K. belliana* is not serrated, or only weakly serrated.

**Acinixys**   This genus contains one species: *Acinixys planicauda*, the Madagascar Flat-shelled spider tortoise. The tail is flattened and its dorsal surface is covered with enlarged scales. There is a slight medial ridge on the maxillae. The plastron is hingeless. The gulars are paired, thickened and extend slightly beyond the rim of the carapace.

**Pyxis**   This genus contains one species: *Pyxis arachnoides*, the Malagasy Spider tortoise. The plastron has a hinge between the humeral and pectoral scutes.

**Chersina**   This genus contains one species: *Chersina angulate*, the South African Bowsprit tortoise. The plastron is hingeless. There is a single gular scute that projects anteriorly. The anal scute is large in contrast to the other species with a single projecting gular scute, *Geochelone yniphora*.

**Homopus**   This genus contains five small species of tortoise. The plastron is hingeless. The gulars are paired, and broader than they are long.

**Psammobates**   This genus contains three species. These colourfully patterned small tortoises are known as South African Star tortoises. The plastron is hingeless. The gulars are paired and broader than they are long. The carapace is domed, with ascending sides.

**Manouria**   This genus contains two species: *Manouria emys*, the Asian Brown tortoise, with two recognised subspecies; and *Manouria impressa*, the Impressed tortoise. The plastron is hingeless. The forefoot has five claws. The supracaudal scute is subdivided into two. Large black blotches occur on the marginal.

**Indotestudo**   This genus contains two species of medium-sized tortoises: *Indotestudo elongata*, the Elongated tortoise; and *Indotestudo forsteni*, the Travancore tortoise. The plastron is hingeless. The forefoot has five claws. The supracaudal scute is subdivided into two. There is a long terminal tail scale. They are a light cream–yellow colour, with brownish blotches on the carapace and to a lesser extent on the plastron. They have a short trachea, which is significant when intubating.

**Geochelone**   This is the largest genus, containing 21 species. All species within this genus are relatively large when adult. The plastron is hingeless. This genus includes the commonly kept species *Geochelone sulcata* (the African Spurred tortoise), *G. pardalis* (the Leopard tortoise) and *G. carbonaria* (the Red-footed tortoise).

**Testudo**   This genus contains six or seven species, depending on whether *Testudo weissingeri* is classified as a species or a subspecies. They all have club-like fore and hind feet. All also have five claws on the forefeet, except for *Testudo horsfieldi*, which has four. The gular scutes are paired, but not projecting beyond the carapacial rim.

- The hinge in the plastron is between the femoral and the abdominal scutes, with the exception of *Testudo horsfieldi*, which lacks the movable hinge.
- *Testudo hermanni* can be distinguished from the others of the genus by having a horny spur on the end of its tail: there are no enlarged tubercles on the thigh and the supracaudal scute is usually divided.
- *Testudo graeca* has an enlarged tubercle on the thigh, the supracaudal scute is undivided and there is no horny terminal tip to the tail. It is important to distinguish the Tunisian tortoise, *Furculachelys nabeulensis*, from *Testudo graeca*. Until recently, it was classified as a subspecies of *T. graeca* due to similarities.

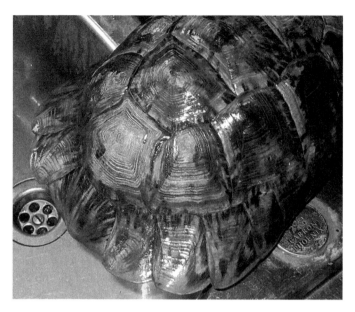

Figure 1.1.1  *Testudo marginata*. Notice the greatly flared supercaudal and posterior marginal.

Unlike *T. graeca*, this species does not hibernate. The key differences from *T. graeca* are as follows: the supracaudal scute is curled; they are very small, with adults rarely exceeding 16.5 cm carapace length; and the carapace is light yellow in colour, with strong black markings in the scute centres. They are brightly coloured: the scutes have a black edging and a black spot in the centre, and there is a distinct yellow spot on the head, between the eyes.

- *Testudo iberia* has a flatter and broader carapace than *T. graeca*. They grow much larger and are often paler in colour, although darker populations do occur. The first vertebral scute is more angular in *T. iberia* compared to the more rounded shape in *T. graeca*.
- In *Testudo marginata*, the supracaudal and the posterior marginal are greatly flared (see Figure 1.1.1). There are four or five longitudinal rows of enlarged scales on the anterior surface of the foreleg.
- *Testudo kleinmanni* is the smallest species (see Figure 1.1.2). There is no tubercle on the thigh, only the supracaudal scute is flared and there are usually only three longitudinal rows of enlarged scales on the anterior surface of the foreleg.
- *Testudo weissingeri* was originally considered a dwarf population of *T. marginata*. They have similar identifying features; however, they are much smaller. They can usually be distinguished from *T. marginata* by the carapace coloration, which is dull brown or blackish, with greyish-yellow or horn-collared patches flecked with grey. This compares with a more contrasting pattern of a pale yellow on black seen with *T. marginata*.

**Gopherus**   This genus contains four species of tortoises from North America. Their forelimbs are flattened as an adaptation for burrowing. The carapace is

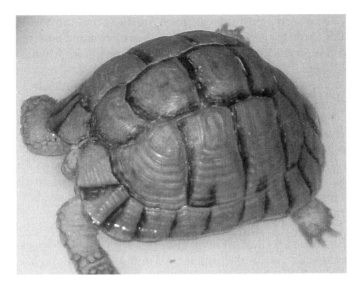

Figure 1.1.2    *Testudo kleinmanni* is the smallest in the *Testudo* genus.

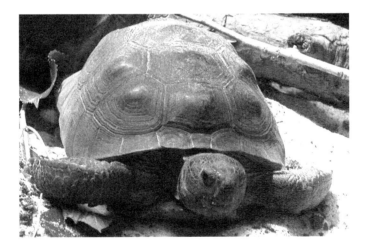

Figure 1.1.3    *Gopherus polyphemus*. Note the lack of a cervical indentation.

flattened and lacks a cervical indentation (see Figure 1.1.3). The plastron is hingeless. They all have paired gular scutes that project anteriorly, especially in males. This genus includes the Gopher tortoise (*Gopherus polyphemus*), which is often kept in North America.

**Malacochersus**    This genus contains one species: *Malacochersus tornieri*, the African Pancake tortoise. The carapace is flattened and flexible. The juvenile carapacial fenestra are retained into adulthood. This allows this species to take refuge in narrow cracks. The plastron is hingeless.

**Emydidae**   These are mainly found in North America. They can be divided between the Box turtles of the genus *Terrapene*, where the anterior and posterior portions of the plastron close completely, and Pond turtles, known in some parts of the world as terrapins, where there is no hinge. The family also includes *Emys orbicularis*, the European Pond turtle, and *Emydoidea blandingii*, Blanding's turtle, where a hinge is present, although in the adult it does not close completely. Inframarginal scutes are absent. There are three or more phalangeal bones in digits 2 and 3 of the hind feet. There is usually some degree of webbing. *Deirochelys reticularia*, the chicken turtle, is recognisable because of its long neck: if measured from shoulder to snout, its length is approximately equal to that of the plastron. *Trachemys scripta elegans*, the Red-eared slider, is instantly identified by the typical reddish marks on the side of its head, often accompanied by a red spot on top of its head. This species is captive farmed in large numbers for the pet trade.

**Geoemydidae**   This is a diverse family of turtles, with about 70 species. It includes the Asian Pond and River turtles, and the Asian Box turtles and other turtles.

**Pelomedusidae and Chelidae**   These are the side-necked turtles. These semi-aquatic animals are carnivorous. Only the Chelidae have a nuchal scute.

## Further reading

Bonin, F., Devaux, B. & Dupré, A. (2006) *Turtles of the World*. A&C Black, London.
Ernst, C.H. & Barbour, R.W. (1989) *Turtles of the World*. Smithsonian Institution Press, Washington, DC.
Ferri, V. (2002) *Turtles and Tortoises*. Firefly Books, Willowdale, Ontario.

# 1.2 Natural History

As with all exotic species kept in captivity, a good knowledge of the natural history of these animals is essential in order to understand their various needs in captivity, especially relating to husbandry, diet, reproduction and behaviour.

The following provides a brief guide to the main species that are kept as pets. As described in Chapter 1.1 and in the sources of information for this section (see below), there is some controversy in the classification and identification of these species. Therefore, some generalisations have been made within these descriptions.

## *Testudo graeca* (Mediterranean Spur-thighed Tortoise)

There is much controversy over the classification of these tortoises. Fortunately, there is much in common between their basic diet and climate.

*Distribution*
*T. g. graeca*, found from northern Morocco to Libya, in southern Spain and in Sardinia/Sicily.
*T. g. terrestris*, found in southern Turkey, Syria, Lebanon, Jordan and from Israel to northern Egypt/Libya.
*T. g. zarudnyi*, found in Iran, Afghanistan and Pakistan.

*Habitat*
Arid areas from sea level to > 3000 m altitude.

*Hibernation*
High-altitude populations hibernate.
Smaller subspecies found at sea level tend not to – they are more likely to aestivate in hot weather. Because of the difficulties in identifying subspecies, smaller thinner individuals should not be hibernated.

*Diet*
Vegetative detritus: a wide variety of fibrous plants, especially their flowers.

*Reproductive data*
- Season: April to June (usually May/June).
- Eggs per clutch: 2–7.

- Laying site: 10 cm deep cavity.
- Incubation time: 3–4 months, although some reports suggest that eggs of *T. g. zarudnyi* may overwinter in the cooler parts of the range.

## *Furculachelys naebulensis* (Tunisian Tortoise)

*Distribution*
Tunisia/western Libya.

*Habitat*
Sea level – arid areas.

*Hibernation*
Does not hibernate.

*Diet*
Vegetative detritus: a wide variety of fibrous plants, especially their flowers.

*Reproductive data*
- Season: April to June (usually May/June).
- Eggs per clutch: 2–7.
- Laying site: 10 cm deep cavity.
- Incubation time: 3–4 months.

## *Testudo ibera* (Greek Spur-thighed Tortoise)

*Distribution*
North-east Greece, parts of the Balkans, the northern Aegean islands, and from parts of Turkey to Iran/Iraq.

*Habitat*
Arid areas from sea level to > 3000 m altitude.

*Hibernation*
From November to February.

*Diet*
Vegetative detritus: a wide variety of fibrous plants, especially their flowers.
However, more omnivorous than *T. graeca*. Some individuals may consume molluscs and insects.

*Reproductive data*
- Season: April to June.
- Eggs per clutch: 6–7.
- Laying site: 10 cm deep cavity.
- Incubation time: 3–4 months.

## *T. hermanni* (Hermann's Tortoise)

*Distribution*
The western subspecies (*T. h. hermanni*) is found in north-eastern Spain, south-east France, western/southern Italy and Majorca, Minorca, Sardinia, Sicily and Corsica.
The eastern subspecies (*T. h. boettgeri*) is found in eastern Italy, the Balkans, Greece and western Turkey.

*Habitat*
Semi-open areas around forested regions.

*Hibernation*
Variable period between October and March.

*Diet*
More than 90% herbivorous – similar to *T. graeca*, but appears to favour legumes and clovers over grasses.
Will opportunistically eat worms, snails and carrion.

*Reproductive data*
- Season: mid-May to July.
- Eggs per clutch: 2–12.
- Laying site: 7–10 cm deep cavity.
- Incubation time: 90 days.

## *T. horsfieldi* (Horsfield's Tortoise, aka Russian/Steppe/ Afghan Tortoise)

*Distribution*
South-eastern Russia, Iran, Afghanistan and Pakistan.

*Habitat*
Dry steppe up to 2500 m altitude.
Usually found near water.

*Hibernation*
Yes – can be > 6 months, as adapted to very hot summers and very cold winters.
Digs long, deep burrows to protect from weather extremes.
May aestivate in summer.

*Diet*
Vegetation – grasses, flowers and leaves.

*Reproductive data*
- Season: mating mid-March to end of April; females lay eggs in May/June.
- Eggs per clutch: 1–5 eggs per nest, in 1–4 nests.
- Laying site: excavated burrows.
- Incubation time: 100 days.

## *T. marginata* (Marginated Tortoise)

*Distribution*
Greece, Sardinia.

*Habitat*
Dry scrub and woodland.
Hillsides.

*Hibernation*
Yes.

*Diet*
Herbivorous – grasses, flowers and some fruits.

*Reproductive data*
- Season: April to June; eggs laid June/July.
- Eggs per clutch: 3–11.
- Laying site: 10 cm deep excavations.
- Incubation time: 2–4 months, depending on soil temperature.

## *T. kleinmanni* (Kleinmann's or Egyptian Tortoise)

*Distribution*
Coastal Libya and Egypt; Israel.

*Habitat*
Desert and semi-desert scrub.

*Hibernation*
No – will aestivate in hot weather.

*Diet*
Mainly herbivorous – especially saltwort and sea lavender.
May take some insects and carrion.

*Reproductive data*
- Season: mating in autumn, with eggs laid in early spring.
- Eggs per clutch: 1 – very large; rarely up to 4.
- Laying site: buried in sand.
- Incubation time: 4–5 months.

## *Geochelone sulcata* (Sulcata or African Spurred Tortoise)

*Distribution*
Sub-Saharan Africa – isolated populations from Mauritania (west) to Ethiopia/
  Eritrea (east).

*Habitat*
Arid acacia forest and woodland.

*Hibernation*
No – will spend dry season in burrows.

*Diet*
Any vegetation.
During the dry season may also take carrion and organic detritus.
Will store dry vegetation in burrows for feeding during the dry season.

*Reproductive data*
- Season: nest November to May.
- Eggs per clutch: 2–4 nestings per female, with up to 19 eggs per nest.
- Laying site: up to 40 cm deep nests.
- Incubation time: 120–210 days, depending on the timing of the rainy season.

## G. *pardalis* (Leopard Tortoise)

See Figure 1.2.1.

*Distribution*
Eastern sub-Saharan Africa and southern Africa.

*Habitat*
Dry savannah, semi-desert, finbos.

*Hibernation*
No, but will hide in tunnels/burrows during cold periods at high altitude.

*Diet*
Mainly herbivorous – almost anything consumed.
Will also take carrion and excrement of other animals.

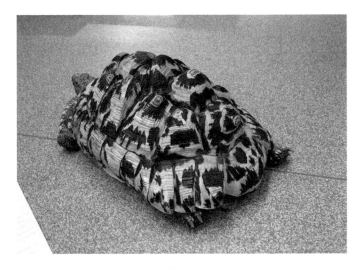

Figure 1.2.1   The Leopard tortoise. Pyramiding may be seen in wild specimens, but is normally a consequence of abnormal growth in captivity.

*Reproductive data*
- Season: warm months – either May to June or October to November, depending on latitude.
- Eggs per clutch: up to 30 eggs each year, in up to six nests.
- Laying site: 10–30 cm deep in dry/stony soil.
- Incubation time: approximately 100 days, but up to 380 days reported.

## G. *carbonaria* (Red-foot Tortoise)

*Distribution*
Northern South America.

*Habitat*
Open areas and dry forest.

*Hibernation*
No – aestivates in summer.

*Diet*
Mainly herbivorous – especially fallen fruit.
Will take carrion and invertebrates.

*Reproductive data*
- Season: June to September.
- Eggs per clutch: 2–15.
- Laying site: against trees, beside pathways in leaf litter or in soil.
- Incubation time: 3–6 months, depending on humidity and sunlight exposure.

## G. *denticulata* (Yellow-foot Tortoise)

*Distribution*
Northern South America and Amazonian lowlands.

*Habitat*
Humid forest – lives under leaves.

*Hibernation*
No.

*Diet*
Insects, larvae and fallen fruit.

*Reproductive data*
- Season: throughout the year with several clutches per female – generally in drier seasons.
- Eggs per clutch: 1–12.
- Laying site: eggs laid on the ground.
- Incubation time: 4–5 months.

## *G. elegans* (Indian Star Tortoise)

*Distribution*
Peninsular India and Sri Lanka.

*Habitat*
Tropical deciduous forest and dry savannah, but does need a supply of water.

*Hibernation*
No.

*Diet*
Herbivorous – especially fruits, vegetables and succulent leaves.
Will eat carrion and insects.

*Reproductive data*
- Season: mates in rainy season; nests May to June and October.
- Eggs per clutch: 3–6 per clutch; up to four clutches per season.
- Laying site: 10–15 cm deep.
- Incubation time: approximately 120 days.

## *Gopherus agassizii* (Desert Tortoise)

*Distribution*
Sonoran and Mojave Deserts in southern United States (USA)/northern Mexico.

*Habitat*
Desert oases, canyon bottoms and rocky hillsides.
Needs sandy/gravelly soil for digging burrows.

*Hibernation*
No, but aestivates for part of the summer.

*Diet*
Largely herbivorous – especially grasses and cacti.
Will also eat carrion.

*Reproductive data*
- Season: nests May to July.
- Eggs per clutch: approximately 6.
- Laying site: 20 cm deep burrow in sandy soils.
- Incubation time: 3 months.

## *Gopherus polyphemus* (Gopher Tortoise)

*Distribution*
Atlantic and Gulf Coastal plains of the USA.

*Habitat*
Well-drained sandy soil between grassland and woodland.

*Hibernation*
No.

*Diet*
Grasses, leaves, hard fruits, bones and insects.

*Reproductive data*
- Season: March to July.
- Eggs per clutch: approximately 7.
- Laying site: often buried close to parent's burrow – approximately 15 cm deep.
- Incubation time: 80–110 days.

## *Trachemys scripta elegans* (Red-eared Slider, or Terrapin)

*T. scripta scripta* may also be seen in captivity – its natural history is very similar to that of *T. s. elegans*.

*Distribution*
South-eastern USA, but has been introduced to many other areas, including the United Kingdom (UK).

*Habitat*
Calm water with a muddy bottom, abundant vegetation and basking sites.

*Hibernation*
Aestivates in summer.
Is capable of hibernation in cooler parts of its range.

*Diet*
Entirely carnivorous when young: older animals also take vegetation.

*Reproductive data*
- Season: courtship in spring/summer, in water; nests on land April to July.
- Eggs per clutch: 2–23.
- Laying site: buried in soil/sand.
- Incubation time: 60–80 days.

## *Terrapene* spp. (North American Box Turtles)

*T. carolina* (Common box turtle) and *T. ornata* (Ornate box turtle) are most commonly seen in captivity.

*Distribution*
USA – the most common species (*T. carolina*) ranges over the entire eastern USA from southern Canada to northern Mexico.

*Habitat*
Mainly wetter woodland close to watercourses.
In dry southern areas, adapts by restricting activity to rainy months and by hiding in mud or under leaves.

Can tolerate salty water, and all species can tolerate periods of weeks to months away from water.

*Hibernation*
Yes – in northern parts of range.

*Diet*
Young mainly carnivorous (invertebrates, carrion), becoming more herbivorous as they get older.
All eat mushrooms.

## *Cuora* spp. (Asian Box Turtles)

The Amboina box turtle (*C. amboinensis*) is most commonly seen in captivity.

*Distribution*
South-East Asia.

*Habitat*
Swamps, small watercourses and rice paddies.
Can also be found on land.

*Hibernation*
No.

*Diet*
Most are omnivorous – the proportion of meat and vegetation varies from species to species.
Young are more carnivorous than older animals.

## Trionychidae (Soft-shell Turtles)

There are a large number of Soft-shelled turtle species – the exact species is often unknown by the owner and the animal's provenance is not always clear.

Where possible, the animal should be identified and its husbandry based on natural history.

*Distribution*
Asia, southern USA, equatorial Africa, Australasia.

*Habitat*
Typical muddy-bottomed streams, rivers, swamps and lakes.

*Hibernation*
No.

*Diet*
Carnivorous, although some species are omnivorous.

## Chelidae (Side-necked/Snake-necked Turtles)

There are a large number of Side-necked turtle species – the exact species is often unknown by the owner and the animal's provenance is not always clear.

Where possible, the animal should be identified and its husbandry based on natural history; however, all species are tropical/subtropical and have similar habitats, meaning that generalisations may be made in terms of husbandry and diet.

*Distribution*
Asia, southern USA, equatorial Africa, Australasia.

*Habitat*
Generally prefer shallow ponds and slow-moving water.

*Hibernation*
No.

*Diet*
Carnivorous, although some species are omnivorous.

## *Carettochelys insculpta* (Fly River Turtle, or Pig-nosed Turtle)

These are often sold to keep in fish tanks, but this is not recommended as they are piscivorous. However, a typical warm-water tank set-up may be appropriate.

*Distribution*
Southern Papua New Guinea and some rivers of northern Australia.

*Habitat*
Calm rivers and lagoon – may also tolerate salt water and enter the sea.

*Hibernation*
No.

*Diet*
Snails, fish crustaceans and fallen fruit.

*Reproductive data*
- Season: nests July to November, in the dry season.
- Eggs per clutch: 15–30.
- Laying site: shallow nests in mud/sand banks – excavated when females emerge from water at night.
- Incubation time: stimulated to emerge by rising water.

## *Chelus fimbriatus* (Mata Mata)

*Distribution*
Northern South America.

*Habitat*
Edges of wetlands and slow rivers.

*Hibernation*
No.

*Diet*
Carnivorous – especially fish and amphibia.

*Reproductive data*
- Season: October to December.
- Eggs per clutch: 12–30.
- Laying site: eroding river cliffs.
- Incubation time: 80 days on average, but varies according to humidity and sun exposure.

# 1.3 Sex Determination and Incubation of Eggs

Determination of sex is not always straightforward in Chelonia. As described below, the vast majority have temperature/environmental-determined sex rather than genetic-determined sex as in mammals and birds.

This means that DNA cannot be used to determine sex (as is done in avian medicine).

In the clinical setting, imaging may be used to visualise the internal gonads: ultrasonography (Chapter 7.2) can be used to visualise mature follicles on the ovary, although coelioscopy (Chapter 7.3) is most useful in visualising and identifying both mature and immature gonads of either sex. However, this technique will require some form of anaesthesia/sedation and is invasive.

Therefore, it is most useful to be able to physically identify sex from the anatomical characteristics of each species. As well as requiring good knowledge of the species involved (see Chapter 1.1), this also requires a lot of experience in determining often subtle differences. Clinicians interested in improving their knowledge are well advised to spend time with experienced breeders of these species and to examine a lot of individuals. This is especially important when trying to sex juveniles, where the differences between the sexes may be minimal. In these cases, it is important that owners are not misled by a 'guess' and uncertainty over the sex of the animal is conveyed to the owner.

Table 1.3.1 gives a brief guide to the different physical characteristics of the sexes in those species covered by this book. Some care is required when using plastron or carapace shape in captive-bred specimens, where abnormal growth and nutritional secondary hyperparathyroidism may affect the shell shape such that the sex-related shape is obliterated.

## Environmental sex determination

As discussed above, in most species (the notable exception being the Soft-shelled turtles, Trionychidae), incubation temperature determines sex. It is, of course, vital to know which temperatures produce which sex offspring if a mixed sex population is to be produced and maintained.

Table 1.3.1 Anatomical sex differences in chelonian species

| Species | | Male | Female |
|---|---|---|---|
| *Testudo graeca* | Mediterranean Spur-thighed tortoise | • Longer, thicker tail; vent opening beyond the rim of the carapace<br>• Concavity of plastron<br>• Wider anal scutes | • Shorter tail; vent opening at, or cranial to, rim of carapace<br>• Flat plastron; some flattening of caudal carapace dorsal to tail<br>• Narrower anal scutes |
| *T. ibera* | Greek Spur-thighed tortoise | • Longer, thicker tail; vent opening beyond the rim of the carapace<br>• Concavity of plastron<br>• Wider anal scutes | • Shorter tail; vent opening at, or cranial to, rim of carapace<br>• Flat plastron; some flattening of caudal carapace dorsal to tail<br>• Narrower anal scutes |
| | <br>Figures 1.3.1 and 1.3.2 Spur-thighed tortoises: male (1) and female (2) | | |
| *Furculachelys naebulensis* | Tunisian tortoise | Longer, thicker tail; vent opening beyond the rim of the carapace | Shorter tail, vent opening at, or cranial to, rim of carapace |

(Continued)

Table 1.3.1 (Cont'd)

| Species | Male | Female |
|---|---|---|
| *T. hermanni* | Hermann's tortoise<br><br>Long tail, with long keratinised tip<br><br><br><br>**Figure 1.3.3** Western subspecies – male | Tail shorter, with shorter keratinised tip |
| | **NB** These differences are very marked in the smaller western subspecies (*T. h. hermanni*). In the larger eastern subspecies (*T. h. boettgeri*), the differences are more subtle. As in the Spur-thighed group (see above), there may be differences in the anal scute. | |
| *T. horsfieldi* | Horsfield's tortoise (aka Russian/Steppe/Afghan tortoise)<br><br>Longer tail, with vent close to the tip | Shorter tail; vent more cranial |
| *T. marginata* | Marginated tortoise<br><br>Longer tail, with vent close to the tip | Shorter tail; vent more cranial |
| *T. kleinmanni* | Kleinmann's or Egyptian tortoise<br><br>Longer tail, with vent close to the tip | Shorter tail; vent more cranial |
| *Geochelone sulcata* | Sulcata, or African Spurred tortoise<br><br>• Anal scute curvature wide and shallow 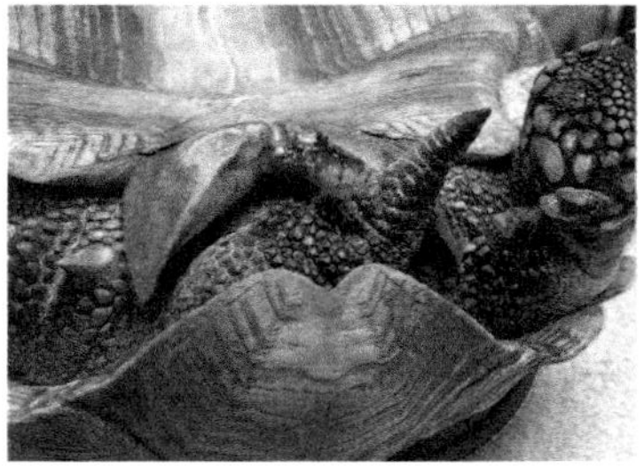<br><br><br><br>**Figure 1.3.5** Note the pointed tail and the shape of the anal scute | • Anal scute curvature deeper and narrower<br>• Plastron flat |

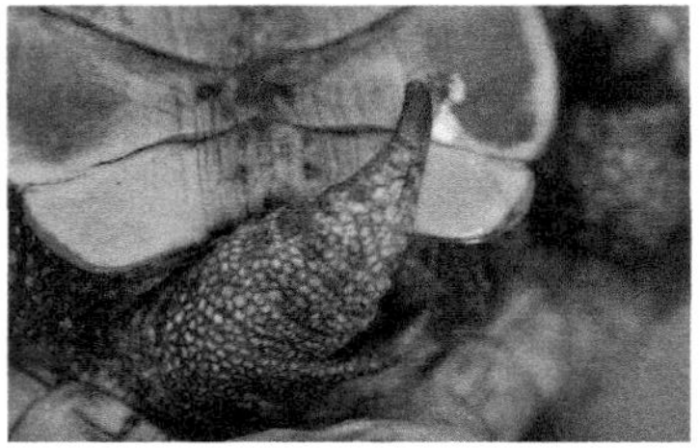

- Plastron concave

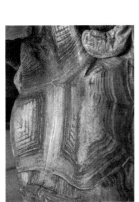

Figure 1.3.6   Note the concave plastron

| G. pardalis | Leopard tortoise | <ul><li>Anal scute curvature wide and shallow</li><li>Plastron concave</li><li>Hindlimb spurs larger in males</li></ul> | <ul><li>Anal scute curvature deeper and narrower</li><li>Plastron flat</li></ul> |

| G. carbonaria | Red-foot tortoise | <ul><li>Longer tail</li><li>Concave plastron</li><li>Anal scute curvature wide and shallow</li><li>'Body shape' thinner, with an obvious 'waist' when viewed from above</li></ul> | <ul><li>Shorter tail</li><li>Flat plastron</li><li>Anal scute curvature deeper and narrower</li><li>Much wider body shape</li></ul> |

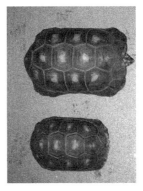

Figure 1.3.4   Male right: female left

| G. denticulata | Yellow-foot tortoise | <ul><li>Concave plastron</li><li>Carapace expanded over hind legs</li><li>Longer tail</li><li>Low, flattened, elongated profile</li></ul> | <ul><li>Flat plastron</li><li>Domed carapace</li><li>Shorter tail</li></ul> |

(Continued)

Table 1.3.1  (Cont'd)

| Species | Male | Female |
|---|---|---|
| G. elegans | Indian Star tortoise | Longer, thicker tail | • Larger than male<br>• Broader profile |
| Gopherus agassizii | Desert tortoise | • Larger than female<br>• Longer tail<br>• Concave plastron<br>• Large glands under chin<br>• Longer claws | • Shorter tail<br>• Flat plastron<br>• Chin glands and claws smaller |
| Gopherus polyphemus | Gopher tortoise | • Concave plastron<br>• Large glands under chin | • Flat plastron<br>• Chin glands much smaller |
| Trachemys scripta elegans | Red-eared slider (or terrapin) | • Smaller than females<br>• Longer tail<br>• Vent caudal to rim of carapace<br>• Some subspecies have long curved claws on forelegs | • Shorter tail<br>• Vent cranial to/level with rim of carapace |
| Terrapene spp. | North American Box turtles | In general, males have longer, thicker tails than the females, with the vent caudal to the carapace rim; some species differences exist in terms of claw length and plastron shape; in the adult common/Carolina Box turtle, the iris is red | In general, shorter tail with vent cranial to/level with the carapace rim; in the adult common/Carolina Box turtle, the iris is yellow–brown |
| Cuora spp. | Asian Box turtles | • Long, thick tail<br>• Concave plastron | • Short, stubby tail<br>• Flat plastron |
| Trionychidae | Soft-shell turtles | Longer tail, with vent near the tip | Shorter tail, with more cranial vent |
| Chelidae | Side-necked/Snake-necked turtles | Longer tail than female; species differences, with some having a concave plastron compared with the female; in some species, the male is flatter than the female | Shorter tail; in some species, the female is more domed than the male |
| Carettochelys insculpta | Fly river turtle (or Pig-nosed turtle) | • Long, pointed tail<br>• Swelling at base of tail<br>• When tail extended, cloacal opening beyond margin of caudal scutes | • Long, pointed tail<br>• No swelling at base of tail<br>• When tail extended, opening just cranial to margin of caudal scutes |
| Chelus fimbriatus | Mata mata | • Longer, thicker tail<br>• Concave plastron | • Shorter tail<br>• Flat plastron |

Table 1.3.2    Temperature-determined sex in Chelonia

| | |
|---|---|
| *Testudo graeca* | Males, 26–29.5 °C |
| *Testudo hermanni* | Mixed, 30–31 °C |
| | Females, 31.5–34 °C |
| *Graptemys* spp. (Map turtles) | Males, 28 °C |
| *Trachemys scripta* (Red-eared slider) | Mixed, 29 °C |
| *Chrysemys picta* (Painted turtle) | Females, 30 °C |
| *Chelydra serpentina* (Snapping turtle) | Females at 20 °C and >30 °C |
| | Males, 22–28 °C |

Table 1.3.2 gives these data for those species where this has been determined (see Deeming 2004).

## Incubation in captivity

In the UK, it is rare that chelonian eggs can be incubated 'naturally', with the possible exception of the temperate freshwater turtles (e.g. the Red-eared slider) in the south of the country. They must therefore be collected and artificially incubated.

Veterinary surgeons are regularly contacted about what to do with eggs that are produced 'unexpectedly'. In these cases, it is essential to check whether the eggs are fertile. In other words, are a male and female both present? This may require sexing of 'parents' (see above).

It is also important to check that the owners actually want to incubate the eggs and possibly hatch offspring. In these cases, they will also need to be advised regarding preparation of vivaria for young Chelonia, and on the legal requirements should they wish to sell or exchange the offspring.

Reptile eggs lack chalazae and are therefore very susceptible to damage when moved. They should always be handled carefully and never turned. Once collected (as soon as possible after laying), they should not be moved again other than for occasional assessment of viability.

Assessment of viability is relatively straightforward in these thin-walled white eggs. Eggs can be candled (as for birds, using a bright light in a dark room) from relatively early in incubation. Because of the difficulty in handling, this is usually only performed near the end of incubation when eggs have not hatched as expected.

The incubation period for most species is not precise and the incubation time will be shorter at higher incubation temperatures. It will also vary slightly according to the surrounding humidity/substrate water content. As an approximation, *Testudo* spp. eggs hatch in approximately 75 days, while softer-shelled freshwater turtle eggs hatch in approximately 55–65 days.

The incubation temperature is influenced by the sex ratio required (see earlier). In general, most breeders try to incubate around the sex determination cut-off temperature unless a very skewed population is required. They have a fairly wide range of tolerance – typically 24–32 °C – though temperatures should be adapted to each species' natural requirements.

Reptile eggs do best in a 'wet' environment. They should be covered in vermiculite or a half sand/soil mixture. They do not need a deep layer of substrate, but should be just covered. In natural conditions, the fluid that accompanies laying will be sufficient to keep the egg moist during incubation. However, when eggs are collected, this is lost. Therefore, the substrate should be slightly dampened after covering. Where the water potential can be assessed, it should be maintained at –150 to –200 kPa. Alternatively, a commercial incubator may be used, with eggs placed on a substrate of damp vermiculite. Water bowls are placed in the incubator such that the humidity is maintained between 50 and 80%.

**NB** Care must be taken with hygiene if doing this, with a safe disinfectant added to the water, coupled with regular changes, in order to avoid bacterial infections.

For more information, see Deeming (2004).

## Reference

Deeming, D.C. (ed.) (2004) *Reptilian Incubation: Environment, Evolution and Behaviour*. Nottingham University Press, Nottingham.

## Further reading

Ernst, C.H. & Barbour, R.W. (1989) *Turtles of the World*. Smithsonian Institution Press, Washington, DC.
Ferri, V. (2002) *Turtles and Tortoises*. Firefly Books, Willowdale, Ontario.
Girling, S.J. & Raiti, P. (eds) (2004) *BSAVA Manual of Reptiles*, 2nd edn. BSAVA, Quedgeley, UK.
Highfield, A.C. (1996) *Practical Encyclopedia of Keeping and Breeding Tortoises and Freshwater Turtles*. Carapace Press, London.
World Chelonian Trust – http://www.chelonia.org/sexdetermination.htm

# 1.4 Physiology/Anatomy

The Chelonia are a subgroup within reptiles.

There are 13 families of living Chelonia, with more than 287 species.

The Chelonia are divided into two groups:

- The Cryptodira, which includes the most commonly seen species. These can draw their heads and necks straight back into their shell.
- The Pleurodira, which bring their heads and necks in to the side (the side-necked turtles).

## The shell

The most distinctive feature of chelonians is their shell. The upper part of the shell is called the carapace and the lower part is called the plastron. They are joined together on both sides by the bridge. The shell is made of about 60 bones fused together. This includes the ribs and most of the vertebrae. The outside of the shell is covered by keratinous scales called scutes: for scute nomenclature, see Figures 1.4.1 and 1.4.2. The margins of the scutes do not line up with the sutures of the underlying dermal bones. Soft-shelled turtles do not have scutes. Instead, their shell is covered with leathery skin. There are numerous variations in the shell shape and the size and number of scutes present. In addition, many species have hinges in their shells. Hinges in the plastron are most common, but a few species have carapacial hinges.

- The pectoral girdle is inside the ribs; that is, inside the shell. The scapula is L-shaped; it meets the humerous and the coracoid bone at its angle to form the shoulder joint.
- The pelvic girdle is composed of the ilium, ischium and pelvic bones, which meet to form the acetabulum. The ilium is attached dorsally to the sacral ribs in the Cryptodira. In the Pleurodira, the pubic and ischium are attached ventrally, giving a more robust framework.
- The limbs are relatively short but contain the same bony arrangement found in the commonly presented mammals; however, there are many modifications

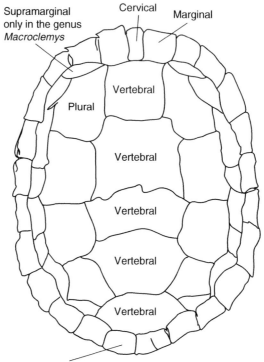

Figure 1.4.1   Carapacial scute nomenclature.

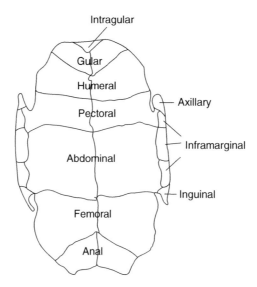

Figure 1.4.2   Plastron scute nomenclature.

of shape. Aquatic species have flattened webbed feet for more efficient swimming.
- The skull is relatively small in most species to allow retraction into the shell. The retractor muscles of the head are well developed to strongly pull the head to safety inside the shell.

## Respiratory system

- Air enters the body through the external nares into the nasal cavity.
- The glottis is located on the floor of the mouth just behind the tongue.
- The glottis is positioned at the choana when the mouth is closed.
- The glottis has two arytenoid and one cricoid cartilages.
- The epiglottis is missing.
- The trachea has complete tracheal rings.
- Tracheal length varies among the species, but in some species it divides into primary bronchi cranially.
- The paired lungs are positioned dorsally against the carapace.
- The lungs are sac-like structures, partitioned into chambers.
- There is no diaphragm. The pleuroperitoneal membrane separating the lungs from the rest of the coelomic cavity is relatively thin and non-muscular.
- Muscle movements of the limbs and the pectoral and pelvic girdles create the negative pressure to draw air into the lungs.
- Chelonians are unable to cough effectively and clear secretions from the lower respiratory tract. This makes recovery from pneumonia more problematic.

See Figure 1.4.3.

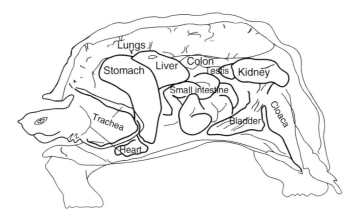

Figure 1.4.3   Anatomy: lateral section.

## Cardiovascular system

- The heart is on the midline, just behind the pectoral girdle.
- The pericardial sac contains a small volume of clear to yellow pericardial fluid.
- The heart is three-chambered, but functionally the pulmonary and systemic circulation are separate.
- There is a renal portal system, but pharmacological trials reveal that the choice of drug injection site does not affect pharmacokinetics.

## Digestive system

### Oral cavity

- Chelonia do not have teeth; they have a horny beak (the rhamphothecae) attached over the jaw bones.
- The lower beak should fit just inside the upper beak, producing a shearing mechanism.
- They will also attempt to rip off pieces of food by retracting their strong neck muscles. In captivity, they learn to put a foot on the food before pulling back.
- Medial to the beak there is a horizontal crushing surface.
- Mucus membranes are moist and have a pink colour.
- They have thick fleshy tongues that have numerous taste buds. Their tongues cannot protrude from the mouth.

### Gastrointestinal section

- The stomach is positioned on the left side, just before the middle of the plastron.
- The small intestines are relatively short and positioned in the caudal half of the coelomic cavity.
- As in most other vertebrates, the small intestines are suspended by the mesentery.
- The small intestine empties into the caecum, which is not well developed.
- The colon can be divided into three parts, the ascending, transverse and descending colon.
- Pebbles and other foreign material often remain in the dilated portion of the transverse colon for prolonged periods. This is on the left side of the coelomic cavity.
- Herbivores have modified the colon into sacculations for microbial fermentation.
- Nematodes of the order Oxyurida are commonly found and are believed to assist in the breakdown of the ingesta.
- The colon terminates in the cloaca.
- The gastrointestinal transit time varies with diet, with the animal in its Preferred Optimal Temperature Zone (POTZ). In herbivorous species, it can vary from 3 to 30 days.

See Figure 1.4.4.

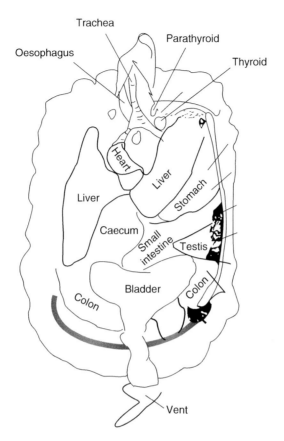

Figure 1.4.4   Anatomy: dorsoventral section.

## Liver

- This large organ is positioned directly posterior to the heart.
- It is divided into two lobes with a gall bladder on the right side.
- The liver's main functions are glucose supply, fat metabolism, fat storage, protein metabolism, blood filtration, bile production and exocrine hormone production.
- Large amounts of fat may be stored in the liver in preparation for reproduction and hibernation.

## Cloaca

- This is a short large bore tube, which terminates through the vent.
- Theoretically, the cloaca is divided into three sections, the coprodeum, urodeum and proctodeum.
- The digestive tract empties into the coprodeum, the proximal portion.

- The genital and urinary tracts terminate in the urodeum, the middle portion.
- These divisions are not very obvious in the animal.

## Urinary system

- The paired kidneys lie in the caudal coelom, just behind the acetabulum.
- The ureters are short and empty into the neck of the urinary bladder.
- The urinary bladder is large. It is a bilobed structure with thin membranous walls.
- The urethra enters the urodeum ventrally.
- Antiperistalsis can move urine anteriorly into the coprodeum and colon, where water can be resorbed.

## Reproductive system – male

- The paired, oval-shaped testis are positioned in the caudal coelomic cavity. They are closely associated with the kidneys.
- The male has a single phallus, which protrudes from the ventral wall of the proctodeum.
- The phallus is not involved in urination. There is a groove – the seminal groove – in the phallus, which can be seen when it is engorged. This transports the semen.

## Reproductive system – female

- There are right and left ovaries, lying just cranial to the kidneys.
- Ovary size varies, depending on the stage of follicular activity.
- Sperm can be stored by the female for several years.
- The oviduct can be divided into five areas, the ostium, aglandular portion, magnum, shell gland and vagina.
- During ovulation, the ostium moves over the ovary to collect the ovulating follicules.
- Follicules pass straight through the aglandular portion to the magnum area, where albumen is added.
- They then move to the shell gland area, where the shell is added.
- Eggs are stored in the vaginal area until deposition.

## Eyes

- Chelonia have functional eyelids and palpebral fissures as found in mammals.
- The lower eyelid is larger and the most mobile, as in birds.
- There is a well-developed nictitating membrane.
- A nasolacrimal duct has not been identified in chelonians.
- Hardarian and lacrimal glands are found in the bony orbit, in similar positions as found in mammals.

- The iris is under voluntary control.
- The retina is avascular, nourished by choroidal vessels.
- The conus papillaris is a vascular structure that projects into the vitreous and is believed to also nourish the retina. It is similar to the pectin oculi of birds.
- Chelonians have both cones and rods, allowing significant colour vision.
- Several species have been shown to have UV vision. Most species of chelonians are believed to have UV vision.

## Smell

- The sense of smell is well developed in chelonians.
- Smell is believed to be an important stimulus to normal feeding.

## Ears

- Chelonia lack an external ear canal.
- The tympanic scale is easily recognised as a circular scale posterior to the eye.
- The auditory canal connects the middle ear with the pharynx.
- The columella, a thin shaft of bone, transfers vibrations from the tympanum to the inner ear.
- The middle ear is divided into lateral and medial sections by an extension of the quadrate bone.
- Chelonians have poor hearing. They only hear low-frequency sounds. Their hearing range is between 50 and 1500 Hz (the low-frequency sounds), compared to the normal human hearing range of 20–20 000 Hz. It is speculated that their ground-borne vibration sensitivity is good; however, this area has not been well studied.

# 1.5   Chelonian Behaviour

As with all captive species, it is essential that normal behaviours are recognised as normal, so that abnormal behaviours can be more readily identified. Many of these may be early warning signs for disease.

Even within those species of Chelonia kept commonly in captivity, there is considerable diversity. As such, this chapter will be a brief overview. For more detailed information, readers are referred to the reading list at the end.

## Aggregation

Chelonian species are not social species. However, aggregation is observed in the field, though in studies of *Gopherus* species it is thought that this only occurs when population densities are high enough. In addition, urine and faeces from 'dominant' males was found to drive some animals away from group sleeping sites.

It is therefore possible to surmise that keeping groups of tortoises together may be stressful to some individuals, especially subordinate males.

## Thermoregulation

All reptiles are poikilothermic – that is, they require external heat supplies and yet are able to regulate body temperature independent of environmental temperature to some degree. It is considered that reptiles tend to exist in a Preferred Optimal Temperature Zone (POTZ), within which they control their core temperature.

Chelonia obtain heat by basking – the carapace has a rich blood supply and a large surface area for this purpose. Therefore, overhead heat sources should be provided. Given that many species are adapted to avoiding excess cold/heat by digging, it seems inappropriate to provide contact heat sources. In addition, the plastron does not appear so well adapted to thermoregulation and prolonged heat mat contact can result in chronic low-grade burns.

Aquatic species (generally, the Soft-shelled species or the Mata mata) will bask in water and will require a shallower water depth under the heat lamp. Semi-aquatic species prefer a shelf or log on to which they can climb to bask.

There appears to be some ability to sense and predict temperature zones. All Chelonia (barring Soft-shelled turtles) have temperature-dependent sex determination, with the sex of the offspring largely being set by environmental temperatures (see Chapter 1.3). There appears to be evidence (certainly within sea turtles) of females selecting nest sites that will result in certain sex ratio skews, depending on the current population pressure. Selection of hibernation sites may also indicate similar abilities.

Many herpetologists believe that sick chelonians (especially those with lower respiratory disease) may, conversely, choose to inhabit the lower end of the POTZ. This would appear to be an attempt to lower the metabolic rate to match the oxygen supply when gas exchange is compromised. Persistent heat avoidance may therefore be an indication of illness. However, this is a short-term survival mechanism that, in the medium to longer term, will compromise the immune response. It is therefore NOT recommended to lower the environmental temperature as part of the therapeutic plan.

Hibernation is a feature of species from temperate zones. The basic stimulus for hibernation appears to be falling temperature. However, there does appear to be some evidence that this response is modified by light cycles. Studies in *Testudo hermanni* appear to show that both exposure to temperatures under 10 °C and light cycles of 16 hours dark/8 hours light were required to reduce both serotonin and melatonin to the low non-cyclical levels seen in hibernation.

## Feeding

Feeding behaviours will vary according to diet.

The herbivorous species tend to forage over large distances, as many are adapted to live in arid/semi-arid areas and fibrous plant material. Care must be taken in captivity not to provide too rich a diet (i.e. succulent foods rich in simple carbohydrates) or obesity/growth deformities may result (see the nutrition section) as fewer calories are expended in seeking food.

When prehending food, many species will smell the food first, appearing to stand over the food and 'huff' (a deep panting breath with movement of the forelimbs – there may be an audible hiss with these breaths). They may then take a light, incomplete bite to 'taste' before beginning to feed properly. In the clinical setting, it is important to recognise these pre-feeding behaviours, especially in the typical anorexic hospitalised tortoise. These behaviours may indicate an animal that is ready to eat, but is not prepared to in the 'hostile' hospital setting. Most will commence eating at home provided that husbandry is adequate.

Diet may vary according to season with some more omnivorous species (e.g. red- and yellow-foot tortoises varying protein consumption between seasons).

Carnivorous species fall into two categories – those that actively forage for food and those that lie in wait for food. In chelonians, the majority fall into the latter category. In the former case (e.g. the Fly river turtle), feeding can be tailored to their activity level, with feeding reduced as the reptile loses interest, in order to avoid obesity and shell deformity.

In the latter case, it is much more difficult to regulate calorie intake to need, as many of these animals appear to be 'programmed' to take food whenever it is presented. Therefore feeding amounts and frequencies must be regulated in conjunction with regular assessment of body condition.

## Drinking

Chelonia do not tend to drink as is understood in mammals – they do not lap or take from bowls/drinkers. All species take water by submersion of all or part of the head and pumping of the throat.

Terrestrial species tend to rely on water from food sources, though this can be unreliable in captivity. Therefore these species should be provided with the opportunity to bath and drink at least once a week.

It is commonly suggested that chelonians also ingest water via the cloaca. While this does occasionally appear to be the case in terrestrial species, it has only been scientifically recorded in aquatic species.

## Social factors

Chelonia are not social species, though they may be gregarious at certain times. Mixing of incompatible species, or of individuals that are very different in size, may result in social 'bullying'.

This may particularly be the case in juveniles, where a larger animal drives the other off food – this can result in an ever-increasing size difference, with the smaller animal failing to thrive and in the larger one selectively feeding and developing shell deformities.

In such situations, the animals may need to be housed separately, either permanently or only at feeding times. A repressed juvenile may continue not to feed adequately if it can scent the presence of the other.

In aquatic carnivorous species, physical damage to the smaller individual may occur. Ideally, all carnivorous species should be fed separately, to avoid the 'feeding frenzy' situation where accidental damage can also occur.

## The circadian cycle

Captive chelonians appear, where possible, to follow daily cycles based on body temperature requirements.

In general, for terrestrial herbivorous species, this will take the following form:

- Bask.
- Feed.
- Bask again – presumably to induce temperatures adequate for fermentation of food in the gut.
- During the remainder of the day, these animals seem able to maintain body temperature by varying behaviours between basking, sheltering from heat and feeding.
- As the temperature drops in the evening, animals will shelter in housing or bury in loose soil.

For carnivorous species, there is some variation. Certainly, they will commence the day basking. However, as they lack the need for fermentation of food, there is no requirement for post-feeding basking.

## Reproductive

### Male

There is little published work on male reproductive cycles. It is thought that chelonian species fall intermediate between androgen-associated and androgen-dissociated cycles of reproductive activity; however, there are no published studies that confirm this hypothesis.

Certainly in captivity, reproductive behaviours can be observed in male tortoises at all times of year if environmental conditions are suitable for metabolic activity.

In terrestrial species, male reproductive behaviours tend to be two phase. The first is visual and involves head bobbing. Eversion of chin glands during head bobbing in *Gopherus* species leads to speculation that the purpose of head bobbing is to release and direct pheromone chemicals.

The second phase is physical. Two males will proceed to ram each other – this may progress as far as overturning the rival.

Where the second animal is female and does not respond by head bobbing, the male will smell the cloacal region and, if identifying female pheromone of the correct species (it is felt that cloacal pheromones are very important in species recognition), will attempt to mate.

In *Testudo* species, there may also be considerable physical stimulation of the female, either ramming (Spur-thighed group) or biting (Hermann's, Marginated and Horsfield's tortoises). It is considered by some that these behaviours may represent a need for ovulation to be induced in the female. In captivity, this has led to considerable shell damage in females of the 'biting' species by male 'rammers' and extensive skin damage to Spur-thighed tortoises by 'biting' males (see Figure 34.4). However, whether this is normal male–female behaviour in an inappropriate setting is not clear. Studies in *Geochelone carbonaria* and *G. denticulata* show that males of one species will rarely attempt mating with females of the other species once they have smelt the cloacal pheromones. It is therefore possible that the aggressive behaviour in captive *Testudos* of different species may represent non-recognition of sex/species and thus attempted male-to-male aggression.

In aquatic species, there may be more elaborate courtship routines. This often involves chasing and scenting of the cloacal region. In some species (e.g. *Trachemys* spp.), the males have long curved claws on the forelegs and these are used to fan the female, presumably to direct pheromone towards her.

### Female

As in males, studies of hormonal regulation in female tortoises are comparatively rare. In *Trachemys scripta elegans*, female reproductive cycles appear linked to oestradiol concentrations.

Female cycles appear to be linked to geographical area, with the dominant factor being temperature variation:

- Winter – metabolic inactivity.
- Spring – rising temperatures linked to follicular growth and vitellogenesis. This parallels spermiogenesis during the same period in males. The female is ready for ovulation in late spring.
- Summer – nesting period. Little follicular growth/activity. In some captive *Testudo* species, females have been observed to become more aggressive in this period.
- Autumn – early follicular growth prior to winter hibernation period.

In tropical species, there appears to be less cyclical activity and breeding timing is less predictable, being based more on food availability, rainfall and so on. Thus mating and egg laying can, potentially, occur throughout the year.

Even in cyclical species, there is potential for autumn mating/egg laying depending on environmental weather conditions. Similarly, there is some confusion between this and the capability of female tortoises to retain eggs for months/years before laying.

Most species held commonly in captivity are nest layers and so require access to adequate areas for this – namely, moderately deep areas of loose substrate. Given the observed ability of females to select nest sites dependent on need and their ability to retain eggs, it is best to provide several such sites in different temperature zones.

## Defensive

Defensive behaviours may take the form of either passive behaviours or active ones.

### Active defensive behaviours

Vocalisation is rare. However, many species (especially terrestrial) may vigorously exhale and hiss when alarmed.

Biting is commonly exhibited by the carnivorous aquatic species. Given the powerful sharp beak, these can cause considerable damage to the handler or to other animals, especially in the larger species.

Terrestrial tortoises may also bite, though this is normally only when a finger is placed on or around the mouth.

Many species (especially aquatic) will scrabble with their legs on being picked up. Damage can occur from the sharp claws.

Terrestrial species may urinate on being handled. Many have large bladders and it is felt that this acts as a water store. However, the manner in which large volumes are forcefully ejected suggests that this water store may also be used as a predator defence.

Given the dual nature of the bladder water store, some authors suggest that a tortoise induced to urinate is given a long bath in order to replenish the water reserve.

### Passive defensive behaviours

The main defensive behaviour is that of retraction into the shell, and all Chelonia are capable of this to greater or lesser extent. Hinging of the shell (in, e.g., box turtles and hinge-backs) can enable complete coverage of the head and limbs when retracted. Otherwise, the hard scales of the distal limbs act to protect the retracted limbs and head. The presence of large sharp spurs on the hind limbs in some species (e.g. Leopard tortoise, African Spurred) can act as an additional defence, and can cause considerable pain if the handler does not release the animal's leg as it is being withdrawn into the shell.

Some semi-aquatic turtle species may release musking agents when alarmed.

## Pain

Reptile pain is poorly understood and poorly described. Basically, any alteration from normal behaviour that occurs after a potentially painful incident (accident, injury, surgery etc.) may be taken as an indication of the reptile feeling pain.

In particular, the following may be used as pain indicators in chelonians:

- anorexia
- resentment of palpation – especially if vigorous and marked on palpating a certain point
- altered posture – raising of body OR dragging
- lameness
- ataxia
- biting at, or rubbing of, a lesion
- withdrawal of one or more limbs or head/tail
- avoidance of other individuals or owner contact
- closed eyes
- reduced activity levels

- neck stretching with or without mouth gaping
- vocalisation – *in extremis*, a screaming sound may be emitted

## Further reading

Gans, C. & Crews, D. (1992) *Hormones, Brain, and Behavior.* Biology of the Reptilia, vol. 18, Physiology E. The University of Chicago Press, Chicago.

Hernandez-Divers, S.J. (2001) Clinical aspects of reptile behaviour. *Veterinary Clinics of North America: Exotic Animal Practice*, 4(3); 599–612.

Kuchling, G. (1999) *The Reproductive Biology of the Chelonia*. Springer-Verlag, Berlin.

Mayer, J. (2006) Reptile behavior. In: *Exotic Pet Behavior* (eds T. Bradley Bays, T. Lightfoot & J. Mayer). Saunders, St Louis, MO.

Petzold, H.-G. (2008) *The Lives of Captive Reptiles*. Society for the Study of Amphibians and Reptiles, Smithsonian Institute, Washington, DC.

# 2 Husbandry

## 2.1 The Husbandry Review

A thorough review of husbandry is an essential part of any chelonian examination. A large proportion of the problems presented are due either directly or indirectly to incorrect or substandard husbandry. The clinician must be familiar with the current best practice for husbandry and nutrition for the species examined.

### Lighting

- Photoperiod – usually 12–14 hours light per day and 10–12 hours dark required.
- UV provision if required – not all species require UVB light. Make sure that the light actually produces the correct spectrum. There is a lot of confusion over the different UV lights available. Many only produce UVA, which is of no use to those species that need a UVB light. Owners are often sold incorrect lights.
- Position – the UVB light must be radiating down on to the basking area, as it is only when it is hitting hot skin that the UV rays are most effective. The distance from the basking area is dependent on the strength of the UVB radiation coming from the light source: too far away and there will not be enough UN radiation; too close and there will be too much. The manufacturer's recommendations on the distance from the basking area should be followed.
- Life expectancy of UV source – the amount of UV radiation gradually deteriorates with time. The rate of deterioration varies with the type of light. As we cannot see UV radiation and the light in the visible spectrum does not vary appreciably, the lights still look the same to us long after the UV output has deteriorated.
- The manufacturer's recommendations on when to replace the light should be followed.

*Essentials of Tortoise Medicine and Surgery*, First Edition. John Chitty and Aidan Raftery.
© 2013 John Chitty and Aidan Raftery. Published 2013 by John Wiley & Sons, Ltd.

- The UV output from a UV light source can be measured. The Solarmeter Model 6.2 UV Meter is the most widely used meter. It is best used to check the ageing of a source. Replace it when the output drops to 70% of the original.
- Do not accept that the lighting is correct: obtain all the lighting details and evaluate whether they are correct. Very commonly, incorrect information is given from apparently reliable sources.

## Thermal provision

- Heat sources – radiant heat from above is ideal, as it mimics the situation in the wild for most species. Heat pads are not recommended, as there are reports in the literature of underfloor heating causing a derangement of gut fermentation, with resultant intestinal rupture and death.
- Thermal gradient – the animal must be able to move between different temperature zones to be able to control its own temperature. There should always be a cool zone.
- Reliability of clients' temperature readings – owners rarely measure the basking area temperature. They will often have a thermometer on the side wall somewhere. Usually, they need to be instructed to move the thermometer to measure the temperatures in the different zones within the enclosure. Many are confused as to how thermostats work. The temperatures that they achieve in the different zones of the environment need to be checked with a thermometer.
- Water temperature – aquatic and semi-aquatic species will have an optimum water temperature range. Some species, especially some turtles of the genus *Trachemys* (e.g. the red-eared slider), can tolerate a wide range of water temperatures; however, they will thrive much better if their water temperatures are within their preferred range.
- Night-time temperature – it is common for night-time temperatures to drop too low. This can cause the animal's body to start the changes that lead to hibernation. Owners will need a max/min thermometer to measure the lowest night-time temperature. This will obviously vary each night. For most species, some form of supplementary heating is required at night.
- The reliability of any temperature control system – no system is completely reliable. There should be at least one thermometer that signals an alarm if the temperature goes above or below the required zone.
- The ambient temperature and the possibility of unplanned temperature spikes – if the sun's rays fall on a vivarium, then the temperature can rocket due to the greenhouse effect. In winter, when the sun is low in the sky, this can happen to vivariums positioned deep in a room.

## Humidity

- Many desert species – for example, *Geochelone sulcata* – need a high humidity microclimate to be available if they are been fed a diet of lush greens that would normally only be eaten by species from more humid areas. This is to prevent pyramiding of the carapace.

- Humidity should not be maintained at the expense of proper ventilation.
- Hygrometers with a remote probe and the display positioned outside the vivarium are recommended, as changes are then more likely to be noticed.

## Enclosure

- Which type; for example, terrestrial, semi-aquatic or aquatic? Is it appropriate for the species?
- Size – is it large enough for the species, ages and numbers?
- Construction material – is it a safe non-toxic material, new or second-hand? If second-hand, could it act as a vector?

## Water quality for aquatic and semi-aquatic species

- Water quality is important for animal health.
- Water should have a low bacterial count and be clear.
- Remove chlorine and chloramine using chemical treatments marketed for fish or by leaving the water standing for 24 hours before the water change (chloramine requires a chemical treatment to remove).
- Removing the animals for feeding will help maintain better water quality, as it reduces food waste and faecal contamination of water (defecation often occurs after feeding).
- Use regular (full changes every 3 days) water changes or filtration to help maintain water quality. Turtles produce a lot of faecal waste, so filtration systems designed for high fish stocking rates are required.
- Normalise the water temperature before putting the animals back in, to avoid a thermal shock.
- A pH between 6 and 8 is suitable for most species.
- Some South American species require a lower pH. Try to replicate the natural environment for the species.
- Aquarium salt can be used to create the brackish-water conditions required by some species – for example, *Malaclemys terrapin*, the Diamondback terrapin from North America.

## Furnishings

- Substrate – many are available commercially. The main criteria are that if ingested, they will not cause an impaction and that contamination with faecal material can be easily removed. Stone slabs as a substrate in part or all of the enclosure are easily cleaned and will keep nails worn down.
- Hides are important in many species. Hides can also provide a high humidity microclimate where needed.
- Plants should not be poisonous if ingested.
- Rocks, if present in the vivarium, should be stable so that they will not roll and injure the animals.

## Hygiene

- How often is the enclosure cleaned and what disinfectants are used?
- What concentration of the disinfectant is used?

## Contact animals

- In-contact animals, including those in the same premises.
- The social structure of the group.
- Breeding history.
- Quarantine protocols for new introductions.

## Nutrition

- Food provided.
- Food consumed.
- Feeding frequency.
- Supplements given.
- Water provision.

### *Common nutritional mistakes*

- Herbivorous chelonia should be fed mainly leafy greens, avoiding all types of lettuce. Lettuce has a low calcium:phosphorus ratio. Fruit and vegetables are normally only an occasional dietary component. If they were a large percentage of the diet, the gut flora of these animals would be unbalanced and they would have to deal with the metabolic changes associated with the more rapid rise and fall of blood glucose levels. There are many negative opinions expressed about complete pelleted foods on the Internet and elsewhere. These diets can produce a more rapid growth rate, so if environmental conditions are not optimum for the species, the more rapid growth will result in deformities earlier than if on a diet producing slower growth rates. A varied diet is advised, where pelleted diets can form up to 50% of the foods fed.
- Omnivorous species such as *Terrapene carolina*, the Common Box turtle, are often fed a diet with a reverse calcium:phosphorus balance of pieces of meat or unsupplemented invertebrates. Ideally, the invertebrates – crickets, mealworms, locusts and cockroaches – should be fed on a proven commercially balanced insect food only. The meat should be replaced with baby mice (pinkies). Fruit, vegetables and leafy greens should also be fed, but avoid the low-calcium items; for example, lettuce, cucumber, bananas, grapes and tomatoes.
- Insectivorous/carnivorous species – most of the aquatic and semi-aquatic species commonly presented are in this group. Meats such as ham, chicken and so on should not be fed, as they are calcium deficient. Whole small mammals and fish are usually readily taken and are a balanced meal. Frozen fish must be

rapidly thawed to reduce the risk of thiamine deficiency. Insects have a poor calcium:phosphorus balance (see above). A varied diet reduces the risk of nutritional problems. Overfeeding is a common problem with these species.

- Commercial terrapin foods that are a mix of freeze-dried invertebrates with pellets, which provide the nutrients missing from the invertebrates, are the most common food associated with nutritional deficiencies. It may be that individual terrapins select their favourite parts of the diet. The commercially available foods, which are all pellets, are rarely associated with nutritional problems.
- Brassicas are often quoted as goitrogenic. This is a theoretical risk: we have seen no clinical cases and none are reported in the literature. In general, to ensure a balanced diet (not because of the risk of goitre), herbivorous chelonians should be fed a varied diet using leafy greens from a range of plant groups.
- Spinach is often incorrectly listed as a plant to avoid. Spinach contains a lot of oxalates, which bind with calcium, making it biologically unavailable. However, there is a lot of calcium in spinach and it still has a lot of biologically available calcium. Many of the plant leaves that form the natural diet are very high in oxyalates. Again, no one ingredient should be fed exclusively. Spinach is a valuable part of a varied diet.
- Fruit – some species, such as *Geochelone carbonaria* (the Red-footed tortoise), are more frugivorous and can be fed a variety of fruits – up to 20% of the diet.
- Hay – many grassland species should have hay as a constituent of the diet. *Geochelone sulcata* (the African Spurred tortoise) and *Geochelone pardalis* (the Leopard tortoise) are examples of species where hay is a normal part of the diet.
- For information on the natural diet, refer to Chapter 1.2.

## Dietary requirements of commonly seen chelonians

There are large variations in the dietary requirements of different species, depending on the ecological niches they have evolved to fill. However, they have been put into nutritional groups for a general overview of dietary needs. Not all species will fit into the general nutritional groups. When the individual species is known, then any variations in its dietary requirements/preferences should be researched.

Water should always be available. It should be deep enough so that the mouth and external nares can be submerged together.

### Plant-based foods
- Requirements vary dramatically between the species. Some require the diet to consist of leafy greens; in others, varying proportions of fruit and vegetables can be provided.
- Always feed a variety of different of foods. Diets based on just one plant species are more likely to be deficient.
- Avoid plants with a negative calcium:phosphorus balance, such as lettuce, grapes, tomatoes, bananas and cucumber.
- Wild-gathered foods can have a high nutritional value.
- Do not wild feed plants that cannot be identified.

- Ensure that wild plants are not gathered from areas that have been treated with chemicals.
- Hay can be digested by only a small percentage of the herbivorous chelonians.
- Most commonly fed fruits have a negative calcium:phosphorus balance and require calcium supplementation.

*Animal-based foods*
- The whole animal is a nutritionally complete package.
- Feeding just part of a carcase results in nutritional deficiencies. For example, when just the meat (muscle) is fed, the phosphorus and protein content is very high and the calcium content is very low, resulting in nutritional metabolic bone disease.
- Whole carcases should be fed. If they are too big, the whole animal can be chopped up so that intake of a balanced diet is achieved.
- Thiamine deficiencies are seen in chelonians fed defrosted fish. Frozen fish should be rapidly thawed and fed immediately. The problem can be avoided by adding a thiamine supplement to the diet, using fresh fish or using a complete formulated diet.

*Insect food*
Many chelonian species are fed insects as part of their diet. The care of the insects has an important influence on their nutritional value:

- If they are going to be a nutritional food themselves, insects must have their own nutritional requirements catered for.
- Insects are deficient in several nutrients, which must be corrected before they are fed.

In additional to other nutritional deficits, insects have a negative calcium:phosphorus balance. This must be corrected before they are fed to the animal. Traditionally, they were covered with a calcium vitamin D dust just before feeding. However, much of this falls off the insect before it is eaten and nutritional metabolic bone disease is frequently seen in chelonians fed dusted insects:

- Insects should be fed a commercially formulated insect food for a minimum of 36 hours before they are used as food.
- Water must also be provided for the insects. A wet sponge or cotton wool sitting in a small container of water that they can reach is adequate. They will drown in shallow water. Providing moist food such as fruit as a water source will result in poor nutrition, as they will then not eat the insect food.
- If not eaten within 2 hours, they should be removed from the chelonian enclosure, as their nutritional value will plummet as the insect food is passed from their gastrointestinal system.

*Commercially formulated diets*
- A wide range of commercially formulated foods are available.
- These have the advantage of convenience.
- Many opinions are expressed about the advantages and disadvantages of using commercially formulated foods.

- There are very few controlled trials published that evaluate the performance of these foods in chelonian species.
- Formulations vary from manufacturer to manufacturer.
- Currently, it is recommended to limit these foods to less than 50% of the diet.
- Choose a brand that has an expiry date, lists the ingredients and provides a nutritional analysis.
- Additionally, ensure that is formulated for that species and life stage.

*Nutritional supplements*
If the diet and environment is correct, then vitamin and mineral supplements are unnecessary.

If fruit consists of greater than 5% of the diet, then a calcium supplement should be given. Follow the manufacturer's recommendations.

Hypovitaminosis A is most commonly seen in semi-aquatic chelonians. They may be unable to convert the beta-carotenes found in plants and need an animal source in their diet.

*Box turtles* (Terrapene *spp.*)
Box turtles are omnivores. Their diet should be approximately 50% animal based and 50% plant based:

- Animal-based foods should be approximately 50% of the diet (more in juveniles):
  - o Invertebrates, crickets, mealworms, slugs, snails and superworms, (the larvae of *Zophobas morio*).
  - o Vertebrates, baby mice (pinkies), whole mice skinned and chopped, goldfish and other feeder fish, fed whole or chopped depending on size.
  - o Dog and cat foods are not recommended.
- Plants should be approximately 50% of the diet (less in juveniles). Fruit can be up to 25% of the diet, with leafy greens and vegetables comprising another 25%. Plant material with a negative calcium:phosphorus balance, such as lettuce (all types), tomatoes, grapes, bananas and cucumber, should be avoided. Very small amounts as treats in an otherwise balanced diet are acceptable:
  - o Fruit – for example, strawberries, raspberries, apples, cherries (remove stone), pears, apples, oranges, peaches, nectarines, mangoes and blueberries.
  - o Leafy greens – for example, the cabbage family (cabbage, kale, Brussels sprouts, cauliflower and broccoli leaves), spinach, pak choi, Swiss chard, parsley, coriander, celery, water cress and rocket. Many weeds that can be gathered from the garden are highly nutritious: common examples are dandelions, plantain, clover, chickweed, docks and sow thistle.
  - o Vegetables – carrots shredded, corn, peas, green beans, bean sprouts, mushrooms, peppers, okra, broccoli florets and chopped squashes.

*Herbivorous tortoises*
*Testudo*, *Geochelone* and *Gopherus* species, among others, are herbivores. There can be a wide variation in dietary requirement between species. For example, the Impressed tortoise, *Manouria impressa*, consumes a diet containing a high

percentage of mushrooms, with fruit and the occasional carrion. In most herbivorous species, the diet should be mainly leafy greens:

- Leafy greens – for example, the cabbage family (cabbage, kale, Brussels sprouts, cauliflower and broccoli leaves), spinach, pak choi, Swiss chard, parsley, coriander, celery, water cress and rocket.
- Wild-gathered plants – common examples are dandelions, plantain, clover, chickweed, docks and sow thistle.
- Vegetables – carrots shredded, corn, peas, green beans, bean sprouts, mushrooms, peppers, okra, broccoli florets and chopped squashes.
- Fruit – for example, strawberries, raspberries, apples, cherries (remove stone), pears, apples, oranges, peaches, nectarines, mangoes and blueberries. Most fruits are deficient in calcium and require supplementation.
- Grasses and hay – some herbivores have the ability to digest grasses and hay. *Geochelone sulcata* and *G. paradalis* both require hay or grass as a major constituent in the diet to prevent accelerated growth and its associated problems.

See Figure 2.1.1.

*Semi-aquatic and aquatic chelonians*
- Most semi-aquatic chelonians are omnivorous.
- Juveniles are more carnivorous.
- Many adults will refuse plant-based foods.
- Vitamin A is required in the diet, as many species may be unable to convert the vitamin A precursors (beta-carotenes) found in plants.
- Whole-body animal-based diets provide vitamin A; otherwise, a supplement should be provided.
- Only healthy prey should be fed; obese, emaciated or diseased prey should be discarded.

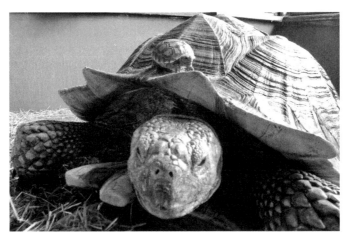

Figure 2.1.1    *Geochelone sulcata* are sold as hatchlings, at which time a correct diet is essential.

- The whole body should be fed. Feeding just meat results in nutritional metabolic bone disease. This will show quickly in rapidly growing juveniles, but may take several years to clinically manifest in adults.
- Edible water plants such as wasabi, water cress, water mimosa and water spinach can be left in the water. Terrestrial plants will affect water quality if not eaten.
- Animal-based foods should only be fed every 3–10 days, depending on the species and age. Juveniles are fed more frequently than adults.

# 2.2   Hibernation

'An extended period of torpor or inertness during the winter months, in which metabolism is greatly slowed down': this is the definition from Elsevier's *Dictionary of Herpetological and Related Terminology*.

The term 'brumation' appears to originate from 1965, when it was proposed as a term for hibernation in reptiles due to proposed differences between hibernation in reptiles and mammals. However, most physiologists reject this separate term, as the specifics of hibernation vary among and within the taxa. However, 'brumation' has achieved widespread use in reptiles, with much confusion over its meaning. It is often mistakenly used when a very ill reptile deteriorates into a state of torpor, with the result that no medical treatment is sought.

It is very important to correctly distinguish between an animal entering hibernation/brumation and one that is ill. Any tortoise described as 'going into hibernation/brumation', especially at the wrong time of the year, should have a full clinical examination, including a review of its environment.

Estivation is a term used to describe a period of reduced activity during hot dry periods in the summer. It is thought to be a strategy to conserve body water employed by turtles in hot arid areas of the world. Tortoises in temperate areas where there are very hot midsummers can also go through a period of estivation; for example, *Testudo horsfieldi* (see Chapter 1.2).

Only species that hibernate in the wild should be subjected to hibernation. Many species are found across a range of environments, where in some areas of the range hibernation is necessary, while there are subpopulations in areas where the environment is such that hibernation is not necessary. For example, in many lowland areas in the southern part of its range, *Testudo gracea* does not hibernate; however, in some of these areas, it estivates due to the very hot midsummers.

The triggers to hibernate depend on the species. Many of the species that normally hibernate, if kept in ideal conditions with no dip in temperatures (day and night) and a constant photoperiod, will stay active through the winter. A few species will stop eating in preparation for hibernation in the autumn, even if the environmental conditions are ideal. This is especially true of mature North American box turtles. In most species, decreasing temperature in the day and/or the night, decreasing photoperiod and reducing food supply are the most important triggers.

## Species that hibernate

Commonly kept species that can hibernate include the Desert tortoises (*Gopherus*); all the genus *Testudo*, with the exception of *T. kleinmanni*; the North American Box turtles of the genus *Terrapene*; the semi-aquatic turtles of the genus *Clemmys*; the American Snapping turtle; and Red-eared sliders (*Trachemys scripta elegans*).

Tropical species such as Red-foots (*Geochelone carbonaria*), Yellow-foots (*Geochelone denticulata*), Elongatas (*Indotestudo elongata*), South American Wood turtles (*Rhinoclemmys*) and the African species do not hibernate, but can slow down for a period of time when the weather cools and the hours of daylight shorten.

In general, there are no hard and fast rules. Most species range over a variety of environments, and there are often subpopulations that, due to their environment, behave differently. For more individual species information, see Chapter 1.2.

## Pre-hibernation evaluation

It is essential that chelonians are healthy prior to hibernation. A pre-hibernation examination is important, as during hibernation there will be significantly reduced capacity to mount a primary immune response:

- Evaluate husbandry and environment for the previous months.
- Weigh and measure (see clinical examination in Chapter 4) to compare with previous date for same individual. This will give a more accurate guide than using Jackson's ratio.
- Carry out a full clinical examination.

Recommended additional testing:

- Ultrasound examination of females' reproductive tract (occult reproductive disease is common).
- Faecal evaluation for internal parasites.

## Preparation for hibernation

In anticipation of hibernation, tortoises need a preparatory period. The most essential aim of the pre-hibernation preparation period is for the gastrointestinal tract to be emptied before hibernation begins. There is evidence that cold conditioning will help them survive lower temperatures. There are many regimes for cold conditioning tortoises for hibernation and gradually reducing their ambient temperatures over 3–4 weeks leading up to hibernation. Warm water baths are often recommended during this period, to stimulate defecation. We recommend the following preparation plan:

- In the first 7–10 days, the tortoise should be maintained at normal vivarium temperatures, be bathed each day and not fed. Night-time temperatures can be allowed to fall to between 10 and 15 °C.

- For the next 7–10 days, the tortoise should be brought down to room temperature, 17–20 °C. The daily bathing is continued.
- For the final 7–10 days, the tortoise may be kept in a garage or outhouse where the ambient temperature is somewhere between 10 and 15 °C, and it should not be bathed or fed.
- It will then be ready to enter the hibernation unit after weighing.

Tortoises naturally hibernate by burrowing themselves in soil deep enough to be safe from the winter freeze. Aquatic species usually hibernate at the bottom of the pond in mud.

An appropriate hibernaculum should be insulated from extreme cold, and be protected from attacks by rodents.

Temperature should be maintained between 4 and 8 °C.

The effect of temperatures below freezing is not completely understood. There are anecdotal reports of vision loss from exposure to sub-zero temperatures, but there are several experimental papers in the literature investigating mechanisms of surviving temperatures below 0 °C. The ability to survive depends on species, size and on whether cold conditioned. We advise keeping the temperature above 4 °C; however, if it falls below this level, many tortoises will wake up unscathed.

If the temperature is higher, the animal will not hibernate properly and will lose weight, leading to depletion.

Some keepers provide a substrate for the tortoise to burrow into.

A fridge as a dedicated hibernaculum will maintain the correct temperatures and facilitate monitoring during hibernation. Many keepers are worried about the theoretical risk of poor ventilation in fridges. Hibernating tortoises require very little oxygen. If worried, keepers can be advised to open the door briefly three times a week to allow an air change. What is important is to keep the fridge in a room where the temperature does not fall below 3–4 °C. The contents of a fridge will freeze if ambient temperatures are below freezing.

It is important that the gastrointestinal tract is empty before cooling to prevent infections secondary to the retention of undigested food. After clearing the gastrointestinal tract, keep the animal at 15–18 °C for a further 4–7 days.

## Hydration

A full bladder and normal hydration status is very important for safe hibernation.

Several warm baths 48 hours apart in the days leading up to hibernation will help with hydration and encourage emptying of the gut.

Place the animal in warm water for 20–30 minutes, up to its chin.

Keep it at room temperature (18 °C) for a further 4–7 days.

## Monitoring hibernation

We advise checking hibernating tortoises every 7–10 days. Weight loss should not exceed 5% for the full hibernation period and is usually much less. A weight loss of 5% or more necessitates ending the hibernation.

Movement in the hibernaculum indicates that the temperature may be too high.

Signs that the animal has urinated denote that the hibernation should be terminated.

### Hibernation length

Normal hibernation lengths vary with the species and the locality. In general, tortoises from more northerly regions hibernate for longer. For most species, a 6–12 week hibernation period is adequate. As a general guideline, it is safer to restrict juveniles for shorter hibernation periods. Hatchlings are best not hibernated, and for yearlings hibernation should be restricted to a maximum of 6 weeks. Many keepers successfully hibernate their tortoises for 4–5 months; however, it is safer to limit hibernation to 3 months in adults.

### Ending hibernation

Temperature is the trigger to emerge. In the wild, on emerging healthy tortoises will bask to bring their body core temperature to normal and start eating within the first day:

1. Remove the tortoise from the hibernaculum.
2. Weigh – a weight loss in excess of 5% may indicate a problem – either a health issue, an incorrect hibernation temperature or the animal has urinated. Most tortoises lose less than 2% of their body weight during hibernation.
3. Check the animal for any signs of disease.
4. Place it in an enclosure at the appropriate temperature, with access to a basking area.
5. Ensure that food and water are available.
6. Monitor appetite, urination, activity and defecation.
7. A healthy tortoise with access to an adequate basking area will start eating on the first day of emergence from hibernation.
8. Animals not eating within 7 days of emergence should be presented for a veterinary examination – earlier if there are any other signs of disease.
9. Warm water baths daily will help the recovery.

# 3 Practice Needs

## 3.1 Equipment

The list here will be in addition to what is found in the typical veterinary practice. Some of the equipment listed below will be available in many primarily dog and cat veterinary practices; however, there are some essential items that will need to be acquired:

- Weighing scales for tortoises – those patients weighing less than 50 grams will require scales that accurately weigh to the nearest 1/10 of a gram.
- Measuring callipers (depending on the size of tortoise).
- An 8 MHz Doppler pencil probe to evaluate the heart and the circulatory system. A flat probe as used for blood pressure measurement can also be used.
- Hospital vivariums equipped with thermostats and the full spectrum of lighting required by most species. Also, for the aquatic and semi-aquatic species there is a need for hospital facilities that can provide a wet area. Water deep enough for swimming is not important for most semi-aquatic chelonians (see Chapter 2.1).
- Intra-osseous catheters or sterile stylets for use with hypodermic needles.
- Tube feeding needles/catheters.
- Specialised surgical requirements (see Chapter 8.1).
- Nutritional support – have a ready stock of elemental diets suitable for the species seen (see Chapter 5.4.1).
- Microchips of small size for chelonians.
- Radiology is essential:
  - Horizontal beam exposure capability is important to image the lungs and will help evaluate if there is a soft tissue swelling deflecting the lungs dorsally.
  - Digital radiography, with its greater processing power, is especially valuable in chelonians. In general with chelonians, it is more difficult to achieve high-resolution images due to the limitations caused by the shell.
- A dremel or similar with appropriately sized grinding stones for burring beaks and nails (see Figure 3.1.1).

*Essentials of Tortoise Medicine and Surgery*, First Edition. John Chitty and Aidan Raftery.
© 2013 John Chitty and Aidan Raftery. Published 2013 by John Wiley & Sons, Ltd.

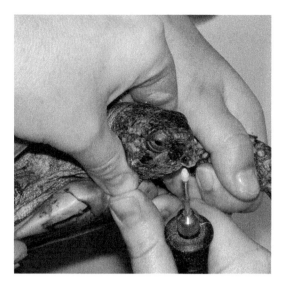

Figure 3.1.1    A burr suitable for use on the beak of a small tortoise.

- Tools for opening the beak and for oral examinations. Dental instruments are very useful in this respect. They are also useful for probing abscesses, wounds and so on.

# 3.2   Economics

Those of us with an interest in tortoises and turtles get great pleasure from helping to promote the health and welfare of these animals. The economics of chelonian medicine is very important, as there are very few who can afford to provide the necessary specialist equipment and the other financial outlays necessary to practice good chelonian medicine without charging realistic fees.

The market for chelonian medicine is much smaller than for the more commonly kept companion animals – that is, dogs and cats – so any investment will take much longer to pay for itself. Most veterinary surgeons work with chelonians because of their special interest in this type of animal, rather than a motivation to increase profit.

## Special requirements

The special equipment is already listed (see Chapter 3.1). Some of this equipment can be used to treat other species, and some may already be available in the veterinary practice, depending on what species is normally treated. Additional costs are as follows:

- Continuing education. As in any other branch of medicine, research and clinical experience bring a continuous chain of clinically relevant information that helps us improve the medical care that we can provide this group of animals. If we are to seriously treat chelonians as opposed to providing emergency care, then it is important to be abreast of the current best standard of care.
- Supporting staff training – in modern medicine, support staff are vital. Their training is an ongoing expense.
- Membership of the Association of Reptilian and Amphibian Veterinarians – the objective of this organisation is to distribute scientific information relating to the field of husbandry, veterinary medicine, and surgery of reptiles and amphibians
- Journal subscriptions. Journals such as *The Journal of Exotic Pet Medicine* and *The Veterinary Clinics of North America Exotic Animal Practice*, in addition to *The Journal of Herpetological Medicine and Surgery*, which comes with membership of the Association of Reptilian and Amphibian Veterinarians, are the most important journals to be reading to stay current in chelonian medicine.
- An up-to-date medical library.
- Reviewing trade catalogues and maintaining pet trade contacts, in order to be aware of developments in the equipment used to provide environmental conditions, and of other products that are becoming available to owners.

## Scheduling appointments

- Initial consultations for chelonians should be scheduled for 20–30 minutes at the minimum.
- Reception training is very important so that receptionists have the knowledge to estimate how long each consultation will take.
- Reception staff need to be able to explain why the longer consultation is scheduled and to justify the charges that need to be levied.
- No-shows are more costly in chelonian medicine, as a longer time is allocated. Many practices have a policy of providing a reminder call on the day before the scheduled appointment.
- Trained support staff can save time by collecting information, biometric data and faecal samples, and by going over changes in husbandry before and after the consultation with the veterinarian.

The practice must be clean, odour free and a pleasant safe place to visit. All staff, and especially the reception staff, must be friendly and knowledgeable. In short, the visit to the veterinary practice must be a positive experience.

## Diagnostic and treatment plans

- The client should be aware that every patient is valued. We should treat all the same, regardless of the monetary value.
- Treatment must be based on the animal's best interests and not its money value.
- Always offer the diagnostic and treatment plan that is in the animal's best interest.
- Always discuss costs.
- Discuss different options, with their advantages and disadvantages.
- Euthanasia should be offered when it is in the best interest of the animal to relieve suffering when appropriate, if the owner is not able or willing to finance treatment, or if treatment is not possible. Seek a second opinion to confirm that there is no possible treatment.
- Offer referral if the case is beyond your level of expertise or equipment.

## Promotion of the practice

- Website – use the practice website to advertise your services and facilities for chelonians.
- Advertise to current clients first: a poster in the waiting room, and a leaflet in with the dog/cat vaccination booster reminders, to make them aware of what you offer.
- A good relationship with a pet shop provides the opportunity to examine and handle healthy animals of less commonly seen species and they may be persuaded to refer their customers to you.
- Practices that do not see chelonians can be a source of new clients.
- Lectures – offering to give talks on chelonian medicine for owners groups, pet store employees and staff from other veterinary practices will help spread the word.

## Advantages for clinicians

- The privilege of working with an amazing group of animals.
- The ability to promote the health and welfare of Chelonia.
- The earliest known Chelonia date from about 215 million years ago – around the time of the start of the dinosaurs – well before lizards, snakes and crocodilian appeared. We have the opportunity to help them survive the effects of mankind.

# 3.3 Hospitalisation

Hospitalisation facilities are essential if chelonians are to be accepted as patients. Many will need to be admitted for sedation to facilitate in-depth examinations or the collection of diagnostic samples. Critically ill animals need to be hospitalised for emergency critical care, and surgical patients will be hospitalised pre and post the surgical procedure.

Ideally, a room should be dedicated as a reptile hospitalisation ward. This should be super-insulated and kept between 20 and 25 °C. Maintaining the ambient room temperature at a higher level makes it much easier to heat individual cages.

If only the occasional chelonian patient is seen, then only one enclosure may suffice if it is equipped so that it can be modified to suit the requirements of different species.

An isolation area is recommended for cases that might have transmittable infectious diseases, so that barrier nursing can be practiced.

All reptile patients should be kept within their individual proper preferred optimal temperature zone.

Treatment plans should be written out in an easily understood form. Tick boxes are good if there are several carers administering the treatment.

## Hospital enclosures

- Non-porous, non-abrasive and easily disinfected are essential requirements.
- Aquariums or large plastic boxes can be improvised as hospital enclosures.
- Humidity, heat and ventilation must be adjustable, based on the needs of the species housed.
- A thermal gradient must be provided for normal thermoregulation.
- Temperatures must be monitored in the hottest and coolest zones by thermometers that are alarmed to alert hospital staff if the temperature moves outside the set limits.
- Night-time temperatures must be controlled and in most species maintained between 20 and 26 °C.
- A basking zone is required by most species where there is visible light and radiant heat, and many also require UVB radiation.

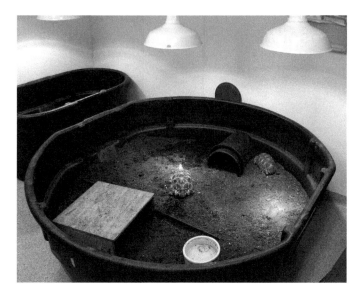

Figure 3.3.1    An improvised hospitalisation environment.

- The photoperiod (night/day cycle) should be similar to that encountered in their natural environment. Where this is unknown, a photoperiod of 12 hours day and 12 hours night can be used.
- Humidity is essential for many species of hospitalised tropical Chelonia. A hydrometer is essential in these cases to ensure that humidity levels are adequate for the given species. For example, *Cuora* species (the Asian Box turtles) require high humidity, whereas *Testudo* species do not.
- Newspaper can be used as a substrate. Any discharges and faecal material passed will be easily seen and collected for disposal or diagnostic testing. It is non-toxic, easily obtainable, cheap and disposable.
- Moribund chelonians will not be able to thermoregulate, so an enclosure with different thermal zones is not appropriate – and can be dangerous, as the animal could become either hyperthermic or hypothermic. A critical care unit where the temperature can be set is ideal. Alternatively, a hospital enclosure can be improvised (see Figure 3.3.1). Ideally, use a water-circulating thermal unit (for zero risk of thermal burns), which is thermostatically temperature controlled to maintain the optimum temperature.
- Visual security is important to some individuals. This can be achieved by providing somewhere to hide, such as under hay or other plant material, or in a small hide box.
- Visual barriers should be provided between enclosures.
- For more detailed information, see Chapter 2.1.
- Hospital charts and identification of the patient should be easily accessed so that observations, such as 'seen eating', and treatments can be quickly recorded.

See also Chapters 1.2, 2.1, 3.3.4, 5.4.1 and 5.6.

### 3.3.1  Dry docking

In veterinary medicine, there are many instances where a smooth recovery requires keeping aquatic and semi-aquatic chelonians out of water. This is called dry docking:

- Aquatic species do better if dry docking can be avoided. If dry docking is essential then maintain in a high-humidity environment, with a minimum of twice daily wound care. They will need to be placed in water for feeding.
- Semi-aquatic species tolerate dry docking better, but often will only eat in water.
- The dry docking period varies with the condition, but can be from days to months as long as there is close monitoring for complications.
- Plastron and bridge lesions may require long periods of dry docking.
- Water intake while dry docked is usually drastically reduced.
- Providing shallow water in bowls may stimulate increased water intake. In some cases, this may have to be reduced to short supervised periods at feeding times. Lesions on the plastron may preclude this approach.
- Fluid intake will need to be supplemented either by the parenteral or enteral route. Aim for a total of 15–25 ml/kg over 24 hours.
- Excretion of faecal material and urates is rarely a problem during dry docking periods.
- Measures to avoid contamination of wounds by faecal material must be taken. Remove faecal material promptly and do not provide any opportunity for climbing, as carapace fractures could be contaminated by the individual falling over faecal material.
- Use a rubber surface if dry docking aquatic species, to avoid plastron lesions.
- Access to water can be phased back in once there is a continuous bed of granulation tissue or if the lesions can be made watertight.

# 3.4   Instructions for Receptionists

Receptionists will be the first members of the veterinary practice to make contact with the owner of the chelonian. They should be trained to recognise urgent cases that need immediate care or refer to somebody within the practice who has the relevant knowledge to make triage decisions. A protocol for organising chelonian appointments should be drawn up. This is in addition to the information normally recorded while making an appointment. The receptionist's protocol for making such appointments should include the following:

- The particular species that the practice has the knowledge and equipment to handle should be recorded.
- Chelonian consultations should only be scheduled for those veterinary surgeons with the necessary knowledge.
- Maintain a list of specialists to whom unfamiliar species can be redirected.
- Request owners to bring in pictures of the environment, in addition to any husbandry records that they keep.
- Require owners to bring in any nutritional supplements and any home remedies that have been used.
- If this is a second opinion or referral, then the previous veterinary history should be obtained and presented to the veterinary clinician as soon as possible.
- Become familiar with the transportation guidelines so that safe advice can be given.

## Chelonian emergency guidance for receptionists

Reptiles have an ability to survive hypoxia for hours. There are reports of chelonians being revived after hours of cardiac arrest. Any chelonian believed to be dead should be checked, as many believed to be dead on initial presentation can be revived with supportive care over hours. Conditions that are emergencies where the animal should be seen immediately are as follows:

- suspected death
- mouth held open and continuously very noisy breathing
- suspected drowning
- haemorrhage
- bite wounds
- shell damage with deficits and coelomic cavity open
- prolapse through the vent
- history of acute trauma

# 4  Examination

## 4.1  Transport Guidelines

- The requirements depend on the ambient temperature.
- As a general rule, keep chelonians at a temperature between 24 and 30 °C.
- On short journeys, a hot water bottle or similar may suffice to keep maintain a suitable temperature within the container. This should be wrapped in a towel to ensure that there is no direct contact between animal and the heat source.
- The ideal transportation container is an insulated box. Polystyrene boxes commercially made for this purpose are available or, alternatively, insulated transport boxes can be improvised from cool boxes.
- Insulated boxes are even more important during hot conditions, to try to prevent the temperature rising above 30 °C.
- Each animal must be transported singly inside a rigid box. Several boxes can be placed inside one insulated container. Cardboard boxes should be avoided.
- Ensure that ventilation is adequate.
- The boxes need to be in an upright position and cushioned to prevent undue movement and jarring.
- They also need to be protected from turning upside down, which could be fatal in a dyspnoeic animal.
- Ideally, a thermometer should be placed in the container so that the temperature can be monitored. This is even more important in hot conditions.
- Thermometers with remote temperature sensors that can be alarmed when they go outside the set limits are ideal.
- The animals must never be left in a car in the sun, as critical temperatures can be reached rapidly.
- When a number of animals are transported together, each should have an identification label.

*Essentials of Tortoise Medicine and Surgery*, First Edition. John Chitty and Aidan Raftery.
© 2013 John Chitty and Aidan Raftery. Published 2013 by John Wiley & Sons, Ltd.

# 4.2 History and Examination Techniques

The previous medical history of the patient and any in-contacts must also be reviewed. This includes treatments carried out by the owner and any previous veterinary treatment.

## Use of questionnaires

- If used correctly, history questionnaires (see Figure 4.2.1) can be very valuable.
- Questionnaires can be made relevant to the species that will be seen.
- A chelonian clinical questionnaire should cover the signalment, source of the animal, in-contact animals, environment, husbandry practices and the nutrition provided for this animal, as well as the symptoms noticed by the owner who initiated the visit.
- It allows relevant parts of the history to be questioned in greater depth.
- It facilitates better use of consulting time.
- It provides an opportunity to evaluate the owner's level of knowledge.

## Physical examination

- It is recommended that the clinician should follow a structured reptile clinical examination and that every patient is examined in the same sequence.
- The clinician must be familiar with what is normal for the species that they are planning to treat. It is only by being familiar with the normal that the clinician will be in a position to recognise the abnormal (see Figure 4.2.2).

### *Observation*

See Figure 4.2.3.

- If possible, observe the animal before handling it.
- Preferably, observe it in its normal housing; however, this is rarely practical and in most cases it will have to be observed in its transport box or on the examination table.
- Allowances have to be made for the effect of any chilling that may have occurred in transit, as this will slow the reptiles down, which may give a misleading impression.

# CHELONIAN HISTORY FORM

Pet name/id............................................ Species.................................................

Sub species..................................................

In present owner's care since............/............/..............

Colour.................................... Date of birth/age..........................................

Sex        Male □   Female □     Unknown □

Where did you obtain this animal?       Breeder □   Pet shop □   Importer □   Other □

Please specify...........................................

## Enclosure/vivarium specifications

Type of enclosure   Terrestrial □   Aquatic □   Environment   Temperate □   Tropical □   Desert □

Size of enclosure        Length................................ Depth....................................

                         Width.............................................

Substrate used..............................................

Temperature daytime range................................Temperature night-time range............................

Day length.........................................

Humidity level        Daytime.................Night-time...................
Method of provision   Spray □   Sprinkler □   Water bowl □

Heating equipment…………………………………..

UV light provision………………… Brand............................................

When was it last renewed?...........................................................

## Diet/supplements

Diet.............................................................................................................................

.....................................................................................................................................

Amount of food normally offered................................ Actually eaten.............................

Frequency of feeding....................................

Method of providing drinking water       Bowl □   Spray □   Other □

Please specify.......................................................................

How often is the water changed?...................................

Vitamin/mineral supplements..............................................................................................

Figure 4.2.1   The chelonian history form.

How are supplements offered?...................................................................................

How often?...............................................................................

**History**

What signs prompted you to bring in this animal?.............................................................

.................................................................................................................................................

Are there, or have there been, any other animals sharing the vivarium in the last 6 months?........

.................................................................................................................................................

Please list any disease history of this animal.................................................................................

.................................................................................................................................................

Please list the disease history of any in-contact animal.................................................................

.................................................................................................................................................

Has this animal been seen by another veterinarian? Yes ☐ No ☐ When?....................

Why?.........................................................

Any other details which may be relevant...........................................................................................

.................................................................................................................................................

**Breeding history**

(please indicate dates of recent attempts at breeding, including changes in temperature, humidity, feeding and animal groupings)

.................................................................................................................................................

Figure 4.2.1 (Continued)

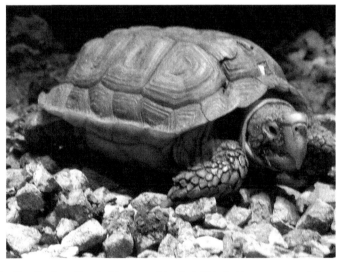

Figure 4.2.2 Familiarity with what is normal is vital. This is *Homopus areolatus* and this beak shape is normal for this species, giving it one of its common names, the Parrot-beaked tortoise.

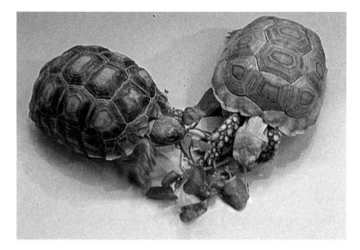

Figure 4.2.3 Colouration can vary between healthy individuals.

- The degree of alertness and general attitude should be observed.
- Locomotion and stance should be studied. Most species ambulate with their bodies held above the ground.
- Eyes should be open and observing the environment.
- Vision.
- Neurological signs such as circling.
- Buoyancy changes to the aquatic and semi-aquatic species (see Chapter 35).
- Nervous individuals will withdraw their heads into the relative safety of their shells.
- The head, if out, should be held up and it should not be resting on the ground.
- Record any limb lameness, weakness or any other abnormal motion observed; also increased or decreased muscle tone, fasciculations and spasm.
- The respiratory rate and effort at rest should be recorded.
- Normally there are no sounds associated with respiration.
- Agitated animals may make hissing noises, which may be mistaken for respiratory infections.
- Open-mouth breathing, gaping, is commonly observed in dyspnoeic animals.

## Measurements

- Weighing is an extremely important part of the physical examination (see Figure 4.2.4).
- The chelonian patient should be weighed at every examination.
- Hospitalised animals should be weighed at the same time every day, ideally first thing in the morning before feeding and bathing.
- Chelonia have large bladders. There can be a large reduction in body weight if the animal has just emptied its bladder, which is a common response to stress.
- Carapace length, width (at the widest part) and height (from plastron bottom to top of carapace) should be measured and recorded to provide a reference in the future for that individual (see Figures 4.2.5, 4.2.6 and 4.2.7).

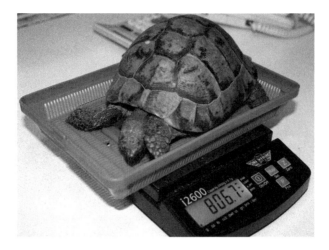

Figure 4.2.4    Recording body weight at each examination is important.

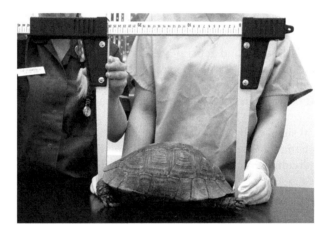

Figure 4.2.5    The straight carapace length.

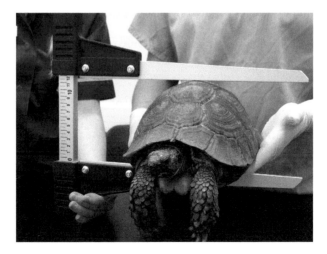

Figure 4.2.6    The carapace depth.

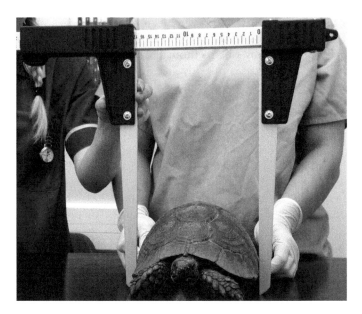

Figure 4.2.7    The carapace width at the widest point.

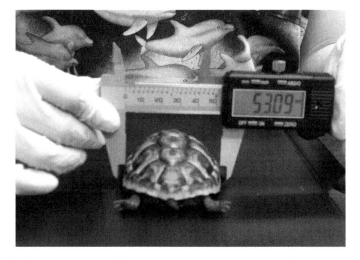

Figure 4.2.8    Using electronic callipers to take measurements in smaller animals.

- Measurements are only useful if there is a historical record for that individual to compare it with or, to a lesser extent, if you have average figures for the species to compare (see Figure 4.2.8).
- Jackson's ratio (Jackson 1980) has been used to assess the body condition of the Mediterranean tortoises *Testudo graeca* and *Testudo hermanni*. The body weight and carapace length are compared to the 'normal' and this used as a

gauge of their health status. However, it is now not used as a measure of health status. There are many reasons why normal healthy tortoises may vary from the 'normal' proposed by this method. There is a great variation between the subspecies and their crosses in body size and shape. The amount of body fat varies through the year. Gut and bladder contents can vary greatly. Additionally, many tortoises in poor condition will fall into the healthy bracket if the Jackson's ratio is used.

- A formula has also been worked out for assessing the body condition of the Californian Desert tortoise, *Gopherus agassizii*, based on the carapace length (*L*), the width at the widest part of the carapace (*W*) and the maximum height from the bottom of the plastron to the top of the carapace (*H*) (Mader & Stoutenberg 1998). Animals weighing less than 90% of the predicted body weight are considered outside their normal range. The predicted body weight = $0.588(L \times W \times H) + 388$. Similar reservations apply to this method as to the Jackson's ratio, but there is less of a body size and shape range in this species.
- These last two methods of assessing body condition must not be applied to other species.

Body condition can also be assessed by palpation, especially if the clinician has experience palpating normal individuals of the species. Emaciation is appreciated by skinny bony limbs, with baggy skin. These individuals are also weak and feel empty when picked up. Overweight individuals deposit fat in the pre-femoral fossa and on either side of the neck. This can be mistaken for oedema (see Figure 4.2.9).

## Clinical examination

Start at the head and work backwards.

Check the rostral areas for abrasions, tissue deficits and any other lesions.

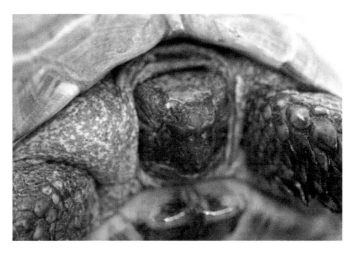

Figure 4.2.9   An obese tortoise.

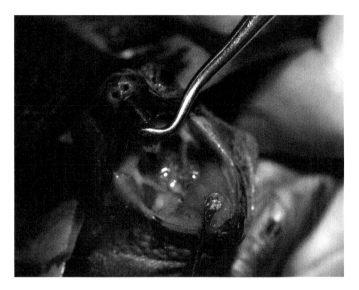

Figure 4.2.10   Oral examination is facilitated by instruments.

## Nares

- External nares should not contain any discharges.
- They should be symmetrical.
- The openings should be patent.
- Using magnification and light depending on the size of the animal, it is possible to see some way in.
- There are no nasal turbinates and no sinuses.
- No dried secretions should be visualised.

## Ears

- In chelonians, the hearing apparatus available for examination is limited. No external ear canal is present.
- A tympanic membrane is present in chelonians. It is caudoventral to the eye. It is seen as a circular scale.
- Bulging of the tympanic membrane is the most common external sign of otitis.
- Occasionally, trauma to the tympanum can cause bleeding or puncture through to the middle ear.

## Oral cavity

- Atraumatic dental instruments may be used to open the beak (see Figure 4.2.10).
- Oral mucus membranes vary from pale to pink in colour.
- Yellowing of the mucus membranes when present is not icterus.
- The choana is the opening that extends anteriorly into the divided nasal chambers.
- Only rudimentary vomeronasal organs are present in Chelonia.
- The beak, tongue and glottis should also be examined at this stage, as explained below.

## Beak

Tortoises are commonly seen with overgrown beaks. Compare the beak of the *Geochelone sulcatas* in Figure 2.1.1 with the beak of the *Homopus areolatus* in Figure 4.2.2. Both are normal for the species.

Lack of wear is a common cause, due to a soft diet. The beak should be growing and being worn down by cutting food at the same rate.

Secondary nutritional hyperparathyroidism can lead to a distorted jaw, leading to overgrowth. Evaluate the shape of the maxilla and the mandible.

Abnormal horn formation can be due to an internal disease process.

Trauma can damage the germinal layers of the beak, resulting in an abnormally shaped beak that would require regular trimming.

See Chapter 5.3.

## Tongue

In chelonians, the tongue is thick, fleshy and has a rough surface:

- The tongue cannot be extended out of the mouth.
- Tongues should be examined carefully for any wounds, abnormal swellings and scarring.
- Glossitis can be seen with a range of viral and bacterial pathogens.
- A whitish-yellow diptheroid membrane on the surface of the tongue, and often involving other surfaces in the oral cavity. Herpesviruses and iridoviruses of the genus *Ranavirus* are important differentials.
- Species, such as Map turtles, that normally eat a lot of hard-bodied prey can develop a crust surface to the tongue if fed soft-bodied prey items.

## Glottis

- The glottis is positioned on the floor of the oral cavity, just behind the tongue.
- It can be difficult to examine. Pressing with a finger between the mandibles while keeping the mouth wide open will bring the glottis into a position where it can be more easily examined.
- Breathing is a two-stage process, consisting of a brief ventilation cycle and a longer pause during which time the glottis is shut. In healthy animals, there can be long intervals between breaths. Rarely there may be a lesion present, which affects the ability of the glottis to open and shut normally.
- A foreign body such as a long hair is occasionally found lodged around the glottis.
- The glottis should be a pink colour, matching the rest of the oral cavity. It should be moist, with no discharges present.
- In cases of respiratory disease, a serous, mucoid or purulent discharge may be seen in and around the glottis and anterior trachea.

- Breathing is normally a silent process. Lower respiratory disease may sometimes cause a wheezing sound on respiration. Discharges in the upper respiratory tract can also make sounds on respiration, but only when the mouth is closed.
- Some tortoises will make a hissing sound when angry.

## Eyes

- Eyelids are present, which can make the ocular examination a challenge. The lower eyelid is bigger and more mobile than the upper.
- Both eyes need to be examined and compared.
- The small eye size makes examination challenging. The use of magnification is essential.
- Inspect the eyelids for any swelling or oedema (chemosis).
- Peri-ocular changes may also be related to ocular disease.
- In a healthy and alert chelonian, the eyes will be open. Also evaluate the eye size for normality. Microphthalmia is seen in chelonians. Exopthalmos is also seen as a result of retrobulbar swellings. Cahexic or dehydrated chelonians can have sunken eyes.
- Chelonia are often presented for keeping their eyes shut. An ocular examination may reveal no abnormalities, as this behaviour is commonly associated with pain from another problem not involving the eyes or associated structures.
- The cornea should be clear, with no deposits, pigments or blood vessels visible. Fluorescein dye can be used to detect any damage to the surface of the cornea.
- The iris pigmentation should be bilaterally symmetrical. Iris colouration is a sexual dimorphism in some species. The iris is striated muscle, so does not respond to mydriatics.
- Under general anaesthetic the iris dilates, allowing the best view of the posterior segment of the eye. Indirect ophthalmoscopy with a 60–90 dioptre lens facilitates examination.

## External body surface

- The entire body surface should be examined visually and palpated. The folds of skin around the cloaca, head and limbs may be especially difficult to visualise, but can be palpated. Familiarity with normal anatomical for the species is essential.
- The skin should be examined for signs of external parasites, wounds, swellings and any colour changes.
- Large skin deficits often heal with scar tissue that is a lighter colour, while dead skin about to slough is a slightly darker colour.
- Reptile skin does not produce blisters in the same way as mammalian skin, due to differences in the vascularity. Burn lesions show up as slightly darker areas of skin. The dead skin may slough several weeks later, revealing a granulating wound.
- Swellings should be assessed for their position, shape, size, whether painful or not, and whether hard or soft.

- Callipers should be used to measure any swellings or areas of discoloured skin where possible.
- Fine needle aspirates or biopsies may be needed to reach a diagnosis.
- Carefully examine areas of dysecdysis and scarring.
- The limbs should be palpated for any swellings that might indicate fractures, metabolic diseases of the bones, areas of osteomyelitis or tumours.
- Missing digits or nails should be recorded, as they may indicate a past infection that may have resulted in bacteraemia, with secondary internal abscesses developing at that time that may now be relevant to the animal's health status.
- Joints should be manipulated to ascertain the range of movement, and the muscles should be assessed for tone and the presence of any twitching that may be caused by nutritional or metabolic conditions, or by toxins.

### Body condition

- Body condition can be assessed by comparing with historical measurements for the individual or, less accurately, with the limitations mentioned above with a normal for the species, in conjunction with the parameters listed below.
- When the animal has lost significant weight, the skin becomes wrinkled and appears too big for the body. Often, the elephantine legs of the species from the Testudinidae feel bony and knobbly and have excess skin.
- The appreciation of poor muscle tone is subjective and comes with experience. An inexperienced clinician can compare with a normal of the same species and size. They will feel weak and floppy when compared with a healthy individual.
- Cachexic tortoises feel empty when picked up and on palpation of the prefemoral fossae they feel hollow.

### Auscultation

- Chelonians are very difficult to auscultate, due to the shell and lack of access to the skin. Doppler blood flow monitors are a much easier way to evaluate heart sounds. A pencil probe is the easiest to use. The probe is placed in the cervicobrachial window and directed towards the heart.
- In individuals with very poorly mineralised plastrons, the probe can be placed on the plastron, just under the heart.
- Auscultation of the lung fields in chelonians is very difficult. The use of a damp cloth under the stethoscope has been recommended. An electronic stethoscope may enhance the lung sounds. Referred sounds from muscle movement commonly interfere with auscultation.
- Aggressive hissing noises must not be confused with abnormal lung sounds.
- A consolidated lung or area of lung will result in a lack of sound over that area.

### Temperature

- Measuring the body core temperature in larger chelonians will be of use in assessing whether the environment provides an adequate temperature. Limitations are the length of time out of its environment and the body size.

Larger chelonians have the ability to slow down their rate of heat loss, so body core measurements in the surgery may give a reflection on the thermal environment provided for them. Reptiles do not increase their body temperatures in response to disease.

- Core body temperature readings are of more value in hospitalised individuals that are not thermoregulating properly, to ensure that they are hospitalised at the correct temperature.

## Coelomic cavity

- Due to their anatomy, chelonians are difficult to palpate.
- The pre-femoral fossae provide windows through which abnormal swellings, such as retained eggs, uroliths and intestinal impactions, may be palpated. Place a digit in each pre-femoral fossa and, holding the tortoise vertically, tilt from side to side. Abnormal swellings are often mobile and may be appreciated bouncing off the finger.
- In larger tortoises, limited digital palpation of the distal coelomic cavity can be accomplished via the cloaca.
- Ultrasound is the best way to evaluate the coelomic cavity.

## Cloaca

- In common with birds and amphibians, the cloaca is a potential cavity into which open the gastrointestinal, reproductive and urinary tracts.
- The vent should be symmetrical and held closed, and should be clean with no discharges present
- Prolapses through the vent are common (see Chapter 31).
- A blunt probe or cotton tip can be used to explore the cloaca. The mucosa should be a normal pink colour.
- No faecal material or urates should be sitting in the cloaca.
- In larger individuals, digital palpation of the cloaca may be possible.
- Probing the cloaca often results in eversion of the phallus. This is normal and gives a chance to evaluate it.

## References

Jackson, O.F. (1980) Weight and measurement data on tortoises (*Testudo graeca* and *Testudo hermanni*) and their relationship to health. *Journal of Small Animal Practice*, **21**, 409.
Mader, D.R. & Stoutenberg, G. (1998) Assessing the body weight of the Californian Desert Tortoise *Gopherus agassizii* using morphometric analysis. *Proceedings of the Association of Reptilian and Amphibian Veterinarians Annual Conference*, 103–104.

# 4.3  Handling

- Wear fresh gloves to handle each individual, unless kept together as a group.
- Wash and disinfect equipment between individuals.
- Do not chill to facilitate handling, as this causes immunosuppression.

## Small to medium-sized tortoises

- Most are not aggressive and are easy to handle.
- Examination can be very difficult if they retreat into their shell. If possible, restraining the forelimbs along the side gives access to the head. Gentle continuous traction will then often facilitate examination of the head. If the head cannot be held, then a blunt probe such as a ball tip seeker can be hooked under the upper beak and gentle traction applied.
- A blunt dental probe or a small spatula can often be slipped in between the jaws to allow visualisation of the oral cavity.
- Some species have functional hinges front and rear and can completely seal themselves into their shell, while others are very strong – and if retreated into their shells, it is very difficult to extend their legs and head out for examination. Sedation is needed in some of these cases. Too much force can injure the animal.
- The animal must be held firmly, as the shell can crack or chip if dropped.
- It can be placed on a pot so that its legs are off the ground to facilitate weighing, radiology and so on (see Figures 7.1.4 and 7.1.5).

## Aquatic and semi-aquatic species

- These species can be very aggressive (e.g. Snapping turtles of the genus *Chelydra*).
- Some can and will give a very serious bite.
- Many can reach their necks a surprising distance, some to the hind legs.
- Sedation is necessary in many individuals.
- The animals will often bite and hold on to a broom handle or other decoy such as a towel or swab on a long forceps, giving an opportunity to move the individual.
- Lift with a hand either side, as far back as possible, or for more aggressive species wrap in a towel.
- Point the head away from assistants and others.

- Some handlers wear heavy protective gloves.
- Do not pick up by the tail or rear limb. They can be quite slippery, so a firm grip is important, as they are easily damaged if dropped.

## Large tortoises – 25 kg or more

- Two assistants are needed to restrain and lift.
- Weighing accurately may be difficult.
- Hospitalisation facilities may be challenging, as because of their size and weight, they often damage walls and their shells.
- Enforced restraint is not possible.
- Many like their head to be scratched, which may facilitate an examination.
- Sedation is often necessary.
- There is a risk of injury to the handler from fingers being trapped by the hinges, between the forelegs or in the pre-femoral fossae when a limb is suddenly withdrawn. It can also be difficult to release a finger trapped in this way.

# 4.4  Zoonoses

Chelonia carry a smaller number of organisms that can potentially cause disease in people, when compared with mammals, due to the fact that they are less closely related to man. Reptiles in general come third in frequency after mammalian and avian zoonosis.

*Salmonella* is the most important reptile zoonosis (see Chapter 9.4):

- *Salmonella* live in the intestinal tract of carrier animals (mammals, birds and reptiles).
- Transmission is by the faecal oral route (usually contamination of food).
- The prevalence of *Salmonella* in chelonians varies widely, depending on the species and the husbandry conditions, with very high prevalence being recorded in semi-aquatic species reared in overcrowded conditions for the pet trade.
- In people, as in reptiles, *Salmonella* can give rise to an unapparent infection, carrier state, enteritis, septicaemia or a combination of these conditions.
- Suspected cases of chelonian to human transmission should have the pathogen serotyped before transmission can be confirmed.
- The elderly, infants and those with impaired immune systems are more at risk.
- Children under the age of five are at an increased risk due to their tendency to put their fingers in their mouths and their lower immunity.
- Useful educational leaflets are produced by the Association of Reptile and Amphibian Veterinarians and Defra (UK).

Mycobacterial infections in Chelonia are rare and it is a very rare zoonosis:

- Cutaneous granulomas may be seen.
- Entry is gained through small breaks in the skin.
- Immunocompromised people may be at a higher risk.

## General hygiene recommendations for reptile owners

- Always wash hands after handling any chelonian, or items potentially contaminated by them.
- Do not keep chelonians in the kitchen, dining room or any food preparation area.

- Never eat, drink or smoke when handling chelonians or their vivaria or associated equipment.
- Immunocompromised people and children less than 5 years of age should avoid contact.
- Vivaria or their furnishings should never be cleaned in the kitchen sink, bathroom sink, shower or bath.
- Always supervise children handling reptiles – their natural inclination to put things in their mouths puts them at greater risk.

# 5    Basic Techniques

## 5.1    Venipuncture and Sample Handling

Given the limitations that the chelonian shell imposes on the physical examination (see Chapter 4.2) and the often non-specific signs with which chelonians are presented, the taking of blood samples is frequently indicated.

Good venipuncture technique and sample handling is essential in ensuring good sample quality and hence better-quality results.

The following gives guidelines on the different venipuncture sites and their advantages and limitations in different species and situations.

### Venipuncture sites

#### *Jugular vein*

See Figure 5.1.1.

*Anatomical landmarks*
There are two branches – dorsal and ventral. The ear scale can be used to locate these branches – the veins run directly along the length of the neck from the dorsal and ventral borders of the ear scale.
The right jugular branches are generally larger than the left.
The veins are very superficial – they may be visualised through the skin such that raising of the vein is not always required.
An 8 MHz Doppler pencil probe device may assist in locating veins.

*Pros*
- 'Gold standard' in terms of sample quality – less chance (though not impossible) of lymph contamination.
- Easy to obtain large samples.
- Possible to catheterise, though difficult to maintain.

*Essentials of Tortoise Medicine and Surgery*, First Edition. John Chitty and Aidan Raftery.
© 2013 John Chitty and Aidan Raftery. Published 2013 by John Wiley & Sons, Ltd.

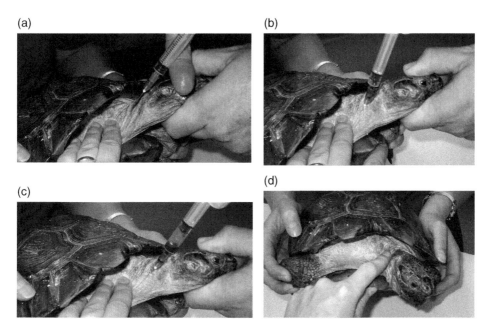

Figure 5.1.1  Venipuncture at the jugular vein. (a) The head is extended and pulled to the left, allowing access to the right jugular vein: the skin is aseptically prepared and the vein raised using digital pressure at the base of the neck. (b) The vein is palpated or visualised and the needle inserted into the vein (it is very shallow). (c) Blood is withdrawn: if lymph is seen, then the procedure should be stopped and restarted. (d) After withdrawal of the needle, firm pressure is applied to the venipuncture site for several minutes to reduce haematoma formation.

*Cons*
- Can be a difficult restraint with large or reluctant individuals.
- Always requires at least two operators.
- The dorsal branch is closely associated with the carotid artery – it is easy to enter the artery inadvertently and cause large haematoma.
- Even if entering the vein directly, prolonged handling may be necessary to avoid haematoma formation.

*Suggested uses*
The jugular vein should be the first choice in all tractable or anaesthetised/sedated individuals.

## Subcarapacial (Subvertebral)

See Figure 5.1.2.

*Anatomical landmarks*
Formed by the anastomosis of common intercostal vessels before joining the external jugular veins.
Located in the dorsal midline, immediately ventral to the spine.

(a)    (b)

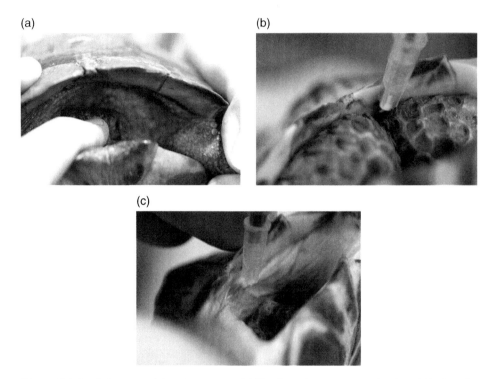

(c)

Figure 5.1.2    Subcarapacial venipuncture. (a) The front legs are restrained and the head is pushed back into the body: the skin dorsal to the head is aseptically prepared. (b) In many tortoises, this vein can still be accessed even if the legs cannot be restrained; however, it is much less easy to locate the correct insertion site or to prepare the skin. (c) A bent needle is inserted where the skin joins the shell in the dorsal midline. The ventral vertebrae are contacted and the needle withdrawn slightly (while applying negative pressure) until blood is withdrawn: if lymph is seen, the needle is withdrawn and the procedure restarted.

A bent needle should be used, entering the midline dorsal to the head where skin joins shell. The needle is angled so as to contact the ventral processes of the spine.

Once the skin is penetrated, negative pressure is applied as the needle is advanced until the vein is encountered.

If the vertebrae are encountered, withdraw the needle slightly.

The head can be restrained in or out of the shell – in the case of aquatic species, it is a good tip to wrap gauze around forceps, allow the reptile to bite this and then gently push the head back into the shell.

*Pros*
- Much easier restraint than for jugular sampling and, in theory, similar samples (size and quality) should be gained.
- Can often be performed by single operator.
- Possible to sample very small individuals.

*Cons*
- Some authors report an increased chance of lymph contamination.

- Some authors report an increased risk of spinal penetration and subsequent haematoma and/or abscess. Thorough skin cleaning is required before venepuncture.
- Long needles may be required in larger individuals, especially *Geochelone* species.

*Suggested uses*
Suitable for all species, though snake-necked turtles may be difficult to restrain.

## Dorsal tail (Dorsal venous sinus)

See Figure 5.1.3.

*Anatomical landmarks*
The dorsal midline of the tail between the spine and the skin, though there is considerable individual variation.
The tail may be sampled when tucked inside the shell, though it is easier to sample if exteriorised and restrained.

*Pros*
- Can be the only accessible vein in some species – especially larger *Geochelone* species.

*Cons*
- Few advantages – high chance of lymphodilution (always inform the laboratory that this is the sampling site).
- Can be difficult to obtain a large sample.
- A difficult area to clean thoroughly, with some risk of introducing infection – the area should be thoroughly scrubbed pre-sampling.

*Suggested uses*
In individuals where it is impossible to sample the jugular or subcarapacial.

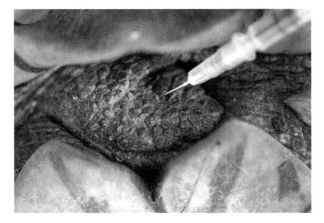

Figure 5.1.3    Dorsal tail vein venipuncture.

### Occipital venous sinus (Dorsal cervical sinus)

*Anatomical landmarks*
The needle is inserted through the skin in the dorsal midline of the neck, just caudal
   to the head.
Direct the needle cranially and slightly laterally, applying negative pressure until
   blood is seen.

*Pros*
- In large individuals, it is possible to get a large sample.

*Cons*
- High probability of lymphodilution.
- Can be a difficult restraint with large terrestrial species.
- Care should be taken in sampling terrestrial species, as ventroflexion of the neck
   may allow needle entry into the spinal cord/hind brain. Due to this risk, it may
   be appropriate only as a route for euthanasia.

*Suggested uses*
In larger individuals, where impossible to sample from other sites.
Euthanasia if other veins inaccessible.

### Brachial/ulnar venous plexus

See Figure 5.1.4.

*Anatomical landmarks*
Extend the front leg.
Palpate the tendon on the caudal (flexor surface) carpal joint.
Insert the needle caudoventral to the tendon, angled towards the joint.

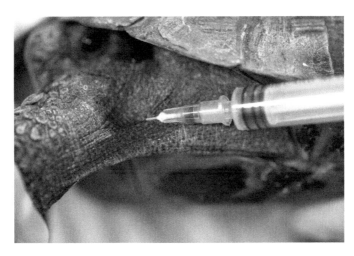

Figure 5.1.4   Brachial vein venipuncture.

*Pros*
- In larger individuals, provides an additional site – can be a very useful site in giant species.

*Cons*
- High probability of lymph contamination.
- Unsuitable for individuals < 1 kg body weight.

*Suggested uses*
Only if impossible to sample elsewhere.
Useful in larger Leopard tortoises/Sulcatas, where only a single limb may be grasped.

## Nail clip

This is not recommended, as contamination with tissue fluid is likely.
There may also be contamination with urine/faeces that will artificially raise the uric acid reading.
Only a small sample is possible.
Sampling will cause pain until the nail heals.

## Heart

*Anatomical Landmarks*
Located immediately dorsal to the plastron, at the midline intersection of the humeral and abdominal scutes (see Figure 5.9.1).

**NB** Hold the animal in 'ventral recumbency' or the heart may fall away from this position.

An 8 MHz Doppler pencil probe device will assist in locating the heart in soft-shelled individuals.

*Pros*
- May enable sampling of very small animals, or where the plastron has not mineralised.

*Cons*
- Possible damage/bacterial contamination of the myocardium, though this is rare. Thorough cleansing of the shell is required before sampling.
- Drilling the shell is likely to cause pain.

*Suggested uses*
Use in juveniles < 50 g if soft-shelled and subcarapacial sampling is unsuccessful.

## Sample size and handling

### Sample size

Up to 3 ml/kg may be obtained from healthy individuals. The maximum sample size should be reduced in sick animals.

## Handling

In general, take blood into heparin tubes – spun gel tubes may be utilised for bio-chemistries (especially electrolytes) if there is to be a delay in processing and the individual is large enough to allow the collection of enough blood.

Some authors recommend collecting blood for haematology in EDTA – most accept that heparin is also suitable. In smaller individuals, it may not be possible to take enough blood for EDTA and heparin.

In very small animals, it may be advisable to use a heparinised syringe for sampling.

In all cases, air-dried fresh blood smears should be made and submitted along with the blood. This negates the risks of blood cell damage due to anti-coagulant.

Before sampling, always contact the laboratory in order to ensure that they are familiar with blood from this species and that the suggested profile fits what is required by the clinician. It is also essential to find out the required volume for testing and anti-coagulant required by the lab, as this may vary according to laboratory preferences and the haematologist's experience.

If in-house equipment is used, assess its suitability for that species, and the ability and experience of the practice haematologist in reading blood smears from chelonians.

Electrolyte, glucose and urea measurements can be very important in the sick chelonian and various in-house machines are suitable for assessing these parameters in chelonians.

# 5.2 Toenail Trimming

In the wild, terrestrial Chelonia spend a lot of time clambering over rocky terrain and digging. They have nails that are harder and longer than the nails of dogs and cats. This gives them a better grip if climbing up a rocky shelf and prevents the nails wearing away too quickly. In the captive environment, they do not wear their nails as fast and overgrown nails are common. However, a high percentage of the requests to trim tortoise nails are unnecessary. Owners are just not familiar with the normal length, or they have got the incorrect impression that it is a procedure that must be done regularly (see Figure 5.2.1).

The captive environment should be arranged to try to reproduce normal wear on the nails:

- Place the food on a large stone slab (preferably not smooth).
- Have different levels in the enclosure, so that the animal has to climb up rocky ledges.
- Exercise outside the enclosure should be on similar surfaces.

In many species of the family *Emydidae* – for example, *Chrysemys picta* (the Painted turtle) and *Trachemys scripta elegans* (the Red-eared slider) – the males have elongated nails on their front toes that play a part in courtship (see Figure 5.2.2).

## Indications for nail trimming

- Overgrown nails.
- To remove a digit from weight bearing due to pathology of the toe.
- To create a clean wound because of trauma to nails (e.g. dog bite injuries).
- Infection of the nail.

### *Invalid reasons for nail trimming*

- Owner's perception that lameness is due to long nails. This is unlikely and would delay a proper investigation of the problem.
- Scratching the floor (if the nails are of normal length, then burring to round off any sharp edges is acceptable).
- Owner getting scratched when picking up the tortoise (see above).

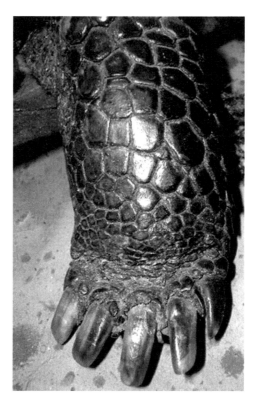

Figure 5.2.1    Note the length of a normal nail and position of the quick.

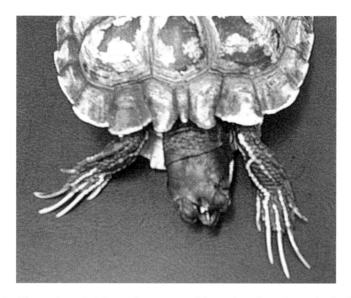

Figure 5.2.2    These elongated forenails are normal for males of most species in the genus *Trachemys*.

## Equipment

- Any nail trimmer that is used for dogs.
- Terrestrial tortoises have very tough nails, so small nail trimmers will not work.
- Use either the pliers type or the guillotine type.
- Use good-quality sharp nail trimmers, as otherwise there is a risk that the nail will be compressed as it is being cut, making the procedure painful and potentially causing damage to the sensitive parts of the nail.
- Bolt cutters may be needed for giant tortoises.
- A rotary power tool such as a dremel is useful to round off any edges or just to file down small amounts of overgrowth. When using a rotary power tool it is important to hold the nail securely.

## Identification of the position of the quick

- On non-pigmented nails, the quick can be visualised as a red area.
- Trans-illumination of the nail, by shining a bright light through the nail, will aid visualisation of the quick in lightly pigmented nails.
- In heavily pigmented nails, identifying the position of the quick is based on experience. There will be individual variation, depending on the length of overgrowth of the nails.

## Nail trimming procedure

- Get an assistant to hold the tortoise.
- Using one hand, hold the appropriate limb.
- Cut the nail to within 2 mm of the end of the quick.
- If there is doubt as to the position of the quick, just remove thin slices of nail (the nail trimmers must be sharp).
- Beware that nails may become projectile missiles; safety glasses may be a good plan.

## Damage to the quick

- If the nail is cut to high up, the quick will be cut. This involves cutting through blood vessels, nerves and bone. If left open, there is the potential for infection to enter the site, which could spread systemically, especially in an already immunocompromised animal.
- Cutting into the quick to collect a blood sample is not considered to be an acceptable technique.
- Cutting into the quick will cause pain and bleeding.
- If a nail is damaged or cut too short, then it should be cauterised and analgesics given. Analgesics can be systemic or local or a combination, depending on the degree of injury.
- Bleeding is the most common sign of quick damage.
- If there is a chronic hepatopathy with a secondary coagulopathy, then bleeding can be excessive.
- Use a topical haemostatic agent and apply pressure directly to the cut surface for several minutes to allow a blood clot to form.

# 5.3 Beak Trim

## Anatomy of the beak

The beak is, essentially, keratin overlying bony ridges. An intervening dermal layer is responsible for continuous growth of the keratin beak.

Given the rarity of beak overgrowth in carnivorous species, it is presumed that the rate of beak growth is much slower in these species compared with herbivorous species whose beaks sustain more wear (see Figures 5.3.1, 5.3.2 and 5.3.3).

As in birds, the beak is comprised of two parts – the upper rhinotheca and lower gnatotheca.

These two parts interact with each other such that each part should wear down the other.

## Causes of beak overgrowth

Essentially, beak overgrowth should not happen unless the dynamic interaction between the two parts of the beak is disturbed. This may be due to altered growth such that the two parts of the beak no longer oppose each other properly, or due to altered keratin synthesis, such that it is not laid down correctly.

Proposed causes of beak overgrowth include the following:

- excess dietary protein and altered growth rate
- nutritional secondary hyperparathyroidism
- vitamin A deficiency
- reduced dietary fibre
- trauma resulting in beak damage
- altered keratin synthesis – secondary to liver disease or dietary deficiency

Beak overgrowth may be a cause of anorexia, as the tortoise is unable to prehend food.

## Methods of beak trimming

It is clear that underlying causes should always be addressed rather than simply trimming the beak. However, in the short term, trimming is essential. The aim of

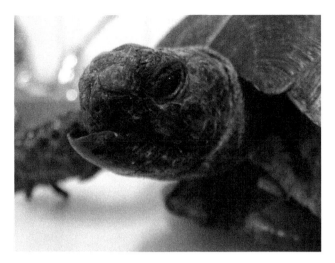

Figure 5.3.1 Overgrown beak in a Spur-thighed tortoise – this situation is typical of cases of metabolic bone disease in early years. Once diet is restored to adequate, the beak often keeps itself maintained in this shape, with only very occasional corrections required.

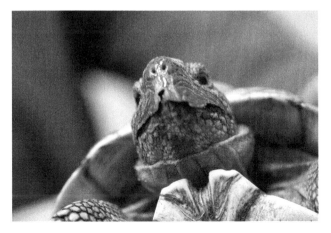

Figure 5.3.2 Overgrown beak in a Red-eared slider – this situation is quite unusual and much less marked than in herbivorous species. Note the irregularity of the lower beak.

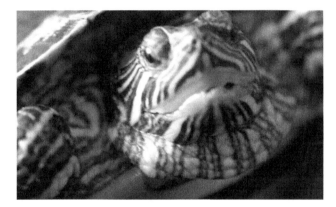

Figure 5.3.3 Overgrown beak in a Sulcata – the keratin is of very poor quality and it is important to investigate underlying causes; for example, liver disease or poor nutrition.

(a)                                         (b)

(c)

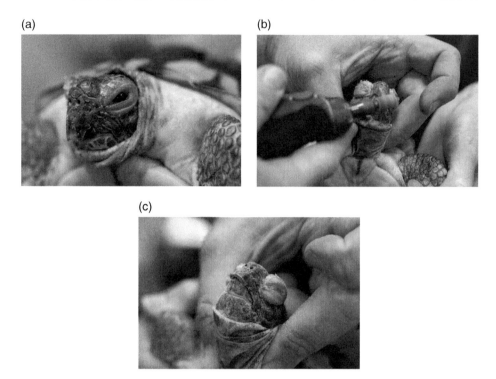

**Figure 5.3.4**   A Hermann's tortoise with beak overgrowth, (a) before, (b) during and (c) after grinding with a motorised tool. Note the need to clean the eyes with damp cotton wool after the procedure in order to remove the fine grinding dust.

this is not simply to reduce beak length but to attempt to restore normal beak anatomy. Therefore, knowledge of different beak shapes in different species is required – for example, serrations seen along the upper beak of Leopard and Sulcata tortoises are not seen in *Testudo* species (see Figure 4.2.2).

Traditionally, trimming has been performed using nail clippers. However, unless done with great care the beak is inclined to split, resulting in damage to underlying structures, haemorrhage and pain.

Ideally, a motorised grinding tool should be used to reshape the beak. In most tortoises, this can be done in the conscious animal – in larger species, sedation may be required (see Figure 5.3.4).

# 5.4 Stomach Tubing

Stomach tubing is a useful way of providing short-term nutritional support. It is to be preferred if the risk of anaesthesia precludes the placement of an oesophagotomy tube. For further information, see Chapters 5.4.1 and 8.3.1.

A specialised feeding tube can be used. These are more commonly marketed for birds and called crop feeding tubes. Alternatively, canine urethral catheters of any other suitably sized catheter that can be attached to a syringe can be used. However, with a canine catheter there is an increased risk of perforation. The feeding tube must be at least the length from the mouth to the middle of the plastron and have a rounded atraumatic end. A protective sheath may be needed in some species – for example, *Trachemys* species (the Sliders) – as they can bite through plastic feeding tubes. Wider-diameter tubes allow easier delivery of the food and should ideally be too large to be accidently passed down the trachea (see Figure 5.4.1).

- Mark the tube at the point where it would be halfway down the plastron.
- Lubricate using a water-soluble, biologically inert lubricant.
- Attach the syringe and fill the tube with fluid to expel the air.
- Hold the chelonian upright. An assistant will be needed to hold the front feet to the side and support the animal upwards.
- Hold the head and draw out to straighten out the sigmoid flexure of the neck. Introduce the tube through the beak and glide it along the roof of the mouth and down the oesophagus, to where it has already been marked.
- Gavage slowly.
- Then withdraw the tube (unless attaching another syringe) and keep upright for a short period afterwards.

This procedure relies on being able to restrain the tortoise. If there is a struggle, consider placing an oesophageal feeding tube. If the animal retracts its head with the tube in position, extreme care is required, as it is possible to perforate the oesophagus due to the sigmoid flexure of the oesophagus in this position.

## 5.4.1 Enteral nutritional support

The aims of nutritional support are to:

- provide an adequate nutritional intake
- prevent the negative effects of malnutrition

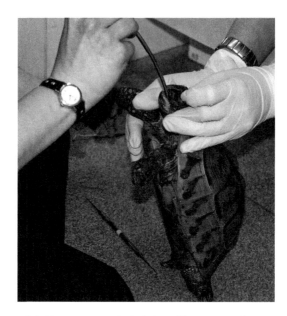

Figure 5.4.1   Stomach tubing an anorexic tortoise with egg retention.

- preserve gastrointestinal structure and function in critical illness
- achieve better outcomes when treating a range of conditions.

Anorexic patients must have nutritional support as part of the treatment plan. There should be a daily reassessment of the patient's changing nutritional needs. Enteral nutritional support is preferable to parenteral nutrition if possible.

Enteral nutritional support can be delivered by stomach tube or by oesophagotomy.

Nasoesophageal, gastrostomy and jejunostomy feeding tubes used in other species are not practical in chelonians due to their special anatomy. Oesophagostomy feeding tubes are the most common mode of nutritional support in critically ill chelonians, as once placed feeding is not stressful and it can be left in for months.

Stomach tubing is the method of choice when:

- nutritional support is going to be short term
- coagulopathies preclude the placement of a oesophagotomy tube
- a high anaesthetic risk precludes the placement of a oesophagotomy tube.

Oesophagotomy tube placement is the method of choice when:

- nutritional support will be needed in the long term
- tube feeding is difficult due to an uncooperative animal
- there is damage/pathology of the head area.

An increased risk of aspiration pneumonia will modify the volumes that can be given. Enteral nutritional support is contraindicated in the presence of gastrointestinal ileus.

## Complications

- Inadequate nutritional intake.
- Intolerance of the food.
- Gastrointestinal dysfunction as a result of enteral feeding can manifest as diarrhoea, ileus or regurgitation.
- Trauma related to the feeding procedure.
- Aspiration pneumonia.
- Metabolic complications; for example, hyperglycemia, the refeeding syndrome.
- Physical blockage of the feeding tube.
- Premature removal of the oesophageal feeding tube.

In the severely dehydrated or very weak patient, the primary aim initially is to rehydrate and restore normal blood pressure. In these cases, if parenteral fluids are not being given, then warmed isotonic glucose saline or other crystalline fluids can be gavaged orally initially to provide a glucose boost, rehydration and some electrolytes. If food is delivered into the gut of patients that may be experiencing inadequate gastrointestinal perfusion, it can lead to mucosal injury and further exacerbate loss of barrier function. Normally, the presence of food in the gastrointestinal tract will result in increased local blood flow. However, in haemodynamically unstable patients, mesenteric blood flow will probably already be compromised and food in the intestine may increase oxygen demand beyond that which can be satisfied by available delivery. This could lead to intestinal ischaemia and loss of barrier function.

Types of nutrition provided can be divided into three different groups:

1. Simple nutritional mixes. These are suitable for very short-term nutritional support. They are not a form of complete nutrition, but are very useful in the acute crisis situation; for example, Critical Care Formula (Vetark, Winchester, UK).
2. Elemental diets are critical care diets that provide liquid nutrients in an easily assimilated form, so that the gastrointestinal tract does not have to work to digest food and has time to heal and begin remission; for example, the Emeraid nutritional care system (Lafeber, Illinois, USA), where the food is provided in three different formulations (herbivore, omnivore and carnivore) that are mixed in different proportions to achieve the correct nutritional balance for the species. After the clinical status improves, most are ready to move to recovery diets. Elemental diets may be fed for an extended period of time in cases of maldigestion/malabsorption. Patients with healthy gastro-intestinal tracts on herbivore or omnivore diets will require more fibre after 7 days.
3. Complete foods in a powdered/liquid format, which can be delivered down a tube. These are sometimes called recovery diets and they require a functioning gastrointestinal tract. This type of food is suitable for long-term nutritional support; for example, Oxbow Carnivore Care and Critical Care (Oxbow, Nebraska, USA), which can be mixed together in different proportions to achieve the correct nutritional balance for the species.

## Indications for enteral nutrition

- Impaired ingestion.
- Inability to consume adequate nutrition orally.
- Impaired digestion, absorption or metabolism.
- Severe wasting or depressed growth.

## Feeding recommendations

- Small volumes frequently.
- Do not exceed the estimated energy requirements.
- Follow the manufacturer's recommendations for the quantity fed and for the dilution factors.
- If the animal is very weak, there will be a risk of aspiration pneumonia. Only give very small volumes or use the parenteral route.
- Only deliver food at the optimum body temperature.
- After prolonged anorexia, give in small amounts – approximately one third of requirements – and gradually build up to the estimated requirements over 4–5 days.
- Reassess requirements daily in the first 7 days.
- Appetite stimulants are not advised, as they will not result in an adequate nutritional intake.

## When to stop nutritional support

- It is a common misconception that while nutritional support is ongoing, the animal will not eat voluntarily.
- As the underlying condition is corrected, the animal's appetite will return and it will show interest in food and begin eating.
- Feedings should not be reduced or suspended solely to check if the appetite has returned.
- The emphasis should not be on appetite, but more on providing nutrients and calories as needed.
- The reduction or stopping of nutritional support is based on an assessment of recovery from the underlying condition.
- Ideally, they should be weaned off nutritional support after discharge from hospitalisation while recovering in their own environment.

The current state of chelonian critical care nutrition is in its infancy, with many extrapolations from mammalian medicine. This is a very important area of critical care medicine, and it is constantly advancing, with new information being published and new products becoming available that open up new possibilities. Important areas needing further evaluation include the optimal composition and the caloric target of nutritional support.

# 5.5 Injection Techniques and Therapeutics

The skin should be cleaned with a suitable disinfectant before any injections. A 10% povodine iodine solution or a chlorhexidine gluconate 4% solution or equivalent are common choices. The needle size is dictated by the medication, but many will easily go through a 29 gauge needle. If the needle has to pass through more than one rubber access diaphragm of multidose vials, then a fresh needle should be attached to the syringe for giving the injection. Many older textbooks recommend that injections should be given in the front half of the body, due to the possibility that drugs given in the posterior part of the may be cleared from circulation by the kidneys due to the presence of a renal-portal shunt. However, pharmacological trials have failed to show any effect on systemic levels of drugs based on the injection site.

## Intramuscular injections

In addition to the above comments, always aspirate after placing the needle to ensure that it is not within a blood vessel before injecting. If fluid is aspirated, then remove the needle and reposition. Switching from side to side between injections will help prevent excessive soreness from repeated injections in the same place.

- Pectoral muscles – this is a good location for intramuscular injections; however, in stronger tortoises access may not be possible. Push the limb laterally and the musculature can be palpated just above the plastron.
- Antebrachial muscles – this site is not recommended if giving an irritant drug such as enrofloxacin, as iatrogenic radial nerve paralysis is common in this site. It can be a useful site in strong individuals where access to other sites is difficult or would require sedation.
- The quadriceps femoris is a common site for intramuscular injections. One hind limb is extended and the quadriceps is the muscle that is palpable proximal to the knee.

## Subcutaneous injections

This site is not as useful as in mammals, due to the poor elasticity of chelonian skin. Some leakage of injected material from subcutaneous sites is common. This site should not be used for irritant substances, as sloughing of overlying skin can occur:

- The pre-femoral fossa. Insert the needle through the skin as far dorsally as possible to reduce leakage from the site.
- The cervicobrachial window, between the neck and the shoulder, is the other site used for subcutaneous injections.

## The epicoelomic space

This is the space between the plastron and the coelomic membrane. The easiest access is between the head and front legs, through the cervicobrachial window. Insert the needle parallel to the plastron. Large volumes can be given in this area and appear to be absorbed relatively quickly.

## The intracoelomic space

Access is via the pre-femoral fossa. It is advisable to position the animal so that it is on its side, with the needle being introduced to the upper pre-femoral fossa. This reduces the risk of perforation of a viscus or rupture of a follicle. Direct the needle towards the ventral half of the fossa, as inadvertent injection into the lungs is easily achieved. Up to 3% of body weight in fluids can be given intracoelomically. Absorption is believed to be slow.

## Intra-osseous catheter placement

This site gives rapid access to the vascular system and is almost equivalent to intravenous injections. Placement of an intra-osseous catheter is a painful procedure, which should be reserved for critical patients. Analgesia should be provided. Intra-osseous catheters, spinal needles or normal hypodermic needles with stylets improvised from orthopaedic wire can be used. The stylet must be pre-sterilised. It needs to be in the needle on introduction to prevent blockage by a plug of bone:

- The bridge between the plastron and the carapace – either an anterior or a caudal approach (see Figure 5.5.1).
- The gular area of the plastron, especially useful in juveniles. There is a large bone marrow space in this area bilaterally.
- The distal ulna – the dorsal tubercle is identified and the needle inserted through this into the medullary cavity.
- The proximal tibiotarsus – the cnemial crest is palpated with the stifle flexed and the needle is inserted slightly on the craniomedial aspect through the insertion of the patellar ligament into the medullary cavity.

## Intravenous injections

See Chapter 5.1.

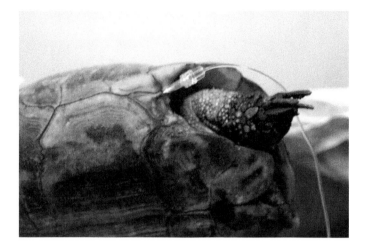

Figure 5.5.1    Intra-osseous access at the bridge.

- Jugular vein – this is the best site for both intravenous injections and blood collection. This is also the site for placement of an intravenous catheter. The jugular runs down the side of the neck, from just behind the tympanic scale. With the head extended, it can often be seen as a linear bulge.
- Subcarapacial blood vessels are used for both blood collection and intravascular injections. Usually the head is pushed into the shell and the skin above the head prepared. A long 25 gauge needle is bent at approximately 30 degrees and introduced at the midline. It is advanced posteriorly and dorsally while maintaining some suction, until the blood vessel in entered. Lymph contamination is common in this area.
- Occipital venous sinus – this site is used in marine chelonians; however, it is not recommended in other species, as spinal cord damage is a possible complication. There are paired sinuses, just lateral to the midline. The head is held in ventroflexion. The needle is inserted behind the occipital protuberance of the skull, just lateral to the midline.
- Brachial vein – this site cannot be visualised through the skin, and sampling is usually blind. Placing a tourniquet at the top of the forelimb will help. Clean the posterior side of one forelimb. Palpate the area, feeling for the triceps tendon. The brachial vein is deep to the tendon. The needle is inserted into the groove at the distal end of the tendon and ventral to the tendon.
- Dorsal coccygeal vein – this site has commonly been used for blood sampling; however, dilution with lymph is common. The skin in this area is often very rough, making sterility difficult. It is a vessel that runs along the dorsal aspect of the coccygeal vertebrae. The tail is extended in a straight line and the needle introduced on the midline.
- Cardiocentesis – this site is most easily accessed in hatchlings with soft shells. The position of the heart can be found with a Doppler pencil probe through the plastron. There are concerns with analgesia on the use of this site (see Figure 5.5.2 and Chapter 5.9).

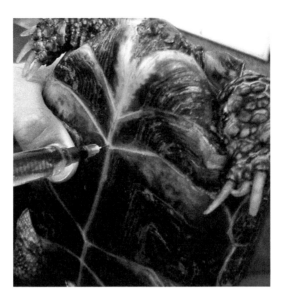

Figure 5.5.2  Intracardiac euthanasia in an anaesthetised animal.

Tortoises have been trained to stretch their heads and hold still for venepuncture (see Weiss & Wilson 2003).

## Topical medication

Topical application of medication is usually reserved for dermatological conditions, with application directly on the lesion. In most chelonian species, the skin presents a thick relatively impermeable layer compared to birds and mammals, so transcutaneous absorption is limited.

## Oral medication

The oral route is a common means of administering medication in chelonians. Liquid preparations are much easier to administer. If it is only a very small volume, then using a syringe to administer it directly into the mouth is usually effective. Large volumes need to be tube fed. If the animal is difficult to tube feed, then inserting an oesophagostomy tube will allow the medication to be administered with minimum stress (see Chapters 5.4 and 8.3.1).

## In-water medication

In-water medication is of no use due to the unpredictable nature of chelonian drinking.

## In-food medication

In-food medication is of use if the animal is still eating. Carnivorous species can have the drug injected into their food items. Herbivorous species can have the medication in fruit. Powdered medications can be folded inside leaves. When using in-food medication, it is advised that where possible the medicated food is hand fed to ensure that it has been eaten. Individuals used to eating pelleted foods can have a batch of medicated pellets made up.

## Reference

Weiss, E. & Wilson, S. (2003) The use of classical and operant conditioning in training Aldabra tortoises (*Geochelone gigantea*), for venipuncture and other, husbandry issues. *Journal of Applied Animal Welfare Science*, **6**(1), 33–38.

# 5.6   Fluid Therapy

Fluid therapy is important in dehydrated animals. Ensuring normal hydration during treatment gives the best chance of recovery. Assessment of dehydration in chelonians is very subjective (see Chapter 9.1). In severely dehydrated individuals, the oral cavity will be tacky, and there may be enophthalmus and decreased skin elasticity:

- If the gastrointestinal tract is functioning, the oral route should be used in preference to parenteral routes. However, in moderate to severe cases of dehydration the parenteral route will need to be used.
- Intravenous catheters can be placed in the jugular vein. A jugular cut-down approach may be required in some cases.
- Epicoelomic fluids are given through the cervicobrachial window into the space just dorsal to the plastron and ventral to the pectoral muscles. Between the foreleg and the head, slide the needle through the skin parallel and just above the plastron. Fluids are rapidly absorbed from this site.
- Intracoelomic fluids are injected into the coelomic cavity via the pre-femoral fossa. Absorption is considered to be rapid from this site. However, there is a risk of rupturing follicles or injecting into the urinary bladder. Hold the animal on its side, so that the organs fall away from the needle, and use the ventral part of the fossa to avoid the lungs.
- Intra-osseous fluids can be given into the gular scutes of the plastron or into the bridge of the shell – either the anterior or the posterior approach.
- Subcutaneous fluids have been described in the pre-femoral fossa and into the skinfold between the neck and the foreleg. However, volumes have to be small due to the inelasticity of the skin – and if peripheral perfusion is poor, absorption will be slow.
- Intracloacal fluids may be administered by giving the fluids via a catheter placed in the distal colon. Bathing will also result in fluid uptake by this route. Bathing of hospitalised chelonians for 10–15 minutes twice daily in water at about 35–37°C will assist in rehydration and encourage emptying of the colon and bladder.

## General principles of chelonian fluid therapy

- Maintenance requirements for chelonians are 10–30 ml/kg per 24 hours.
- Blood volume in healthy reptiles varies from 4% to 8% of body weight, which is 40–80 ml of blood per kilogram.

- Approximately 70% of body fluid is intracellular (in mammals, intracellular fluids account for approximately 60%).
- Chelonians can withstand larger blood losses than mammals or birds, due to their ability to compensate for hypovolemia by transferring fluid from the intra-cellular space.
- They can compensate for dehydration to some degree by resorbing fluid from the urinary bladder.
- Ongoing losses – for example, diarrhoea – should be allowed for in the calculation.
- Deficits should be corrected over 24–72 hours, depending on the level of the deficit, more severe deficits being corrected more slowly.
- Chelonians tend to have the lowest blood pressure (15–40 mmHg) of reptiles. Mammalian or avian parameters of fluid therapy based on blood pressure measurement will result in excessive fluids being administered and subsequent tissue oedema.
- Fluids administered should be warmed to the mid-temperature of the preferred optimum temperature for the species before administration.
- Serial urea and uric acid level measurements will help evaluate the response to fluid therapy.

## Fluids

- Crystalloids such as glucose-saline can be given as a continuous infusion intra-osseously or intravenously, or given in boluses of 5–10 ml/kg. It can be given in larger boluses by any of the other parenteral routes.
- Hypertonic fluids should not be used, as hypovolemia is usually compensated for by shifting fluid between the interstitium and the intravascular compartments.
- Isotonic fluids are best.
- Lactate is often listed as an ingredient that should be avoided in reptiles. This is a controversial opinion. However, it is safer to avoid lactated fluids in severe hepatopathies.
- Colloids are used to expand plasma volume. Both natural and synthetic colloids are used in chelonians. They must be given intra-osseously or intra-venously.
  - o  Synthetic colloids – for example, Haemaccel (MSD Animal Health, UK) – are more economical to use than the alternatives. However, they do not transport oxygen to the tissues. Availability and cost are major advantages when compared with whole blood, plasma or oxyglobin. They are usually combined with crystalloids in a continuous infusion or can be given as boluses at 3–5 ml/kg.
  - o  Oxygen-carrying colloids – for example, oxyglobin – have the advantage of being readily available for use in emergencies, having a colloid effect in addition to being a potent carrier of oxygen. Their main disadvantage is cost. There have been no clinical trials to establish safe dose rates; however, oxyglobin has been used in chelonians at boluses of 5 ml/kg repeated up to a total of 20–30 ml/kg, apparently without adverse effects.

    o  Blood transfusions have not been reported in chelonians. No information about blood groups is available and there are no studies on blood transfusions in the literature. There would be a high risk of spreading disease. They cope surprisingly well with low haemocrits as long as the condition has developed chronically.

# 5.7 Cytological Sampling and Biopsy

Cytology is a powerful tool in veterinary medicine. It is easy to perform, cheap and gives rapid results. In terms of suspected bacterial infections, it can be deemed more sensitive than bacteriology as, not only is it possible to detect bacteria that do not grow easily in laboratory culture, but the body's cellular response is also seen.

It also has the advantage of being relatively non-invasive and can frequently be performed in the non-anaesthetised animal.

The following techniques may be used.

## Impression smears

Indicated for ulcerated lesions, especially mouth lesions (all species) and skin lesions in aquatic species. Some attempt should be made to remove obvious surface contamination or samples should be taken pre- and post-scraping or cleaning. If non-diagnostic or further sampling is required, excisional or pinch biopsies may be taken under sedation/anaesthesia.

## Fine needle aspirates (FNA)

Suitable for all masses, whether solid or liquid-filled. Some care should be taken with these, as many tortoise masses and inspissated abscesses are poorly exfoliative, so non-diagnostic samples may be obtained. It is also important to remember that FNA sampling is a means of collecting cells and the sample collected will not give an indication of the architecture of the lesion. This reduces the diagnostic capability of this technique. Its great advantage, however, is that it is relatively non-invasive and so can be performed in the conscious animal, provided that the lesion is accessible. Otherwise, 'Trucut' (under sedation and/or local anaesthesia) or excision (part or complete under general anaesthesia) may be performed (see Chapter 22).

## Joint tap

In all cases of swollen joint(s) – see Chapter 36. The insertion site should be prepared aseptically. A 21–25G needle (depending on size – use the largest bore that can be safely used) is inserted into the joint space and fluid aspirated.

## Washes

These are appropriate for problems in cavities, especially the lungs.

Lung wash is indicated in cases of generalised diffuse pneumonia and may be performed in the conscious animal (terrestrial species) as long as it can be physically restrained. In very large terrestrial species or aquatic species (due to risk of biting the tube), sedation will be required.

The following technique may be utilised:

- Use the Jackson cat catheter – the diameter depending on the size of the animal. In giant species, use the dog urinary catheter. If worried, a mouth gag may be inserted so that the animal does not bite down and sever the plastic catheter.
- Open the mouth and direct the catheter into the glottis – if possible, towards the lung most clearly affected (as indicated by radiographs).
- Insert saline at a rate of 5 ml/kg.
- Inject and aspirate saline several times – when injecting, raise the head above the level of hindquarters and vice versa when aspirating.
- A 10% yield of fluid is a good yield.
- Submit part for bacteriology (swab or fluid in a plain tube).
- Submit the rest for cytology –
  - o fluid in EDTA plus one drop formol-saline
  - o air-dried smears

## Stains

Cytological smears are prepared as per other species.

Several smears should be prepared per sample and the following stains may be used:

- Plain slide – especially in joint aspirates, an air-dried unstained slide should be examined for the presence of gout tophi (these may be washed off by staining techniques). Ideally, polarised light should be used.
- Trichrome stain – for example, 'Diff Quik' (Dade) – for cellular identification and detection of bacteria/fungi.
- Gram stain – identification of bacteria.
- Ziehl–Nielson stain – for identification of mycobacteria. This should be used for all solid or granulomatous lesions, or for ulcerated skin lesions in aquatic species.

### Further reading

If performing in-house cytology, good reference texts or atlases should be used. The following can be recommended:

Campbell, T.W. & Ellis, C.K. (2007) *Avian & Exotic Animal Hematology & Cytology*, 3rd edn. Blackwell, Oxford.

Campbell, T.W. & Grant, K.R. (2010) *Clinical Cases in Avian & Exotic Animal Hematology & Cytology*. Wiley-Blackwell, Oxford.

Wilkinson, R. (2004) *Clinical Pathology in Medicine and Surgery of Tortoises and Turtles*. (eds S. McArthur, R. Wilkinson & J. Meyer). Blackwell, Oxford.

# 5.8 Microchipping

Microchipping provides a permanent form of identification. In the European Union, it is a legal requirement for all CITES Annex A species (e.g. *Testudo* species other than *T. horsfieldi*) over 10 cm carapace length that are on public display, that are to be sold or exchanged, or that are breeding offspring for sale/exchange.

Internationally, see http://www.cites.org for a list of national contacts and information of local enforcement of the CITES regulations.

Current UK guidance may be found on the Defra website at http://www.defra.gov.uk and it is important to consult this before advising on any legal aspects of permanent identification of Chelonia, especially when dealing with novel species or live animal exports.

The following, from the Defra website, gives the basic advice for CITES identification:

*Marking for tortoises*

To qualify for a specimen-specific certificate, live Annex A tortoises must be marked with an unalterable microchip that meets ISO Standards 11784:1996 and 11785:1996 (E). If this is not possible due to the physical or behavioural characteristics of the specimen concerned, they must be marked with a uniquely-numbered band, tag, tattoo or other appropriate method. We will record the identification number and marking method on the certificate issued for that specimen. You must get appropriate advice from your vet to make sure that the marking is carried out by taking account of the humane care, wellbeing and natural behaviour of the specimen.

We recognise that tortoise hatchlings under 100 millimetres long (from one end of the shell to the other) are too small to be safely fitted with a microchip, so we can issue transaction certificates for these specimens. However, these certificates are no longer valid if the tortoise is not microchipped when it reaches 100 millimetres long and a condition in box 20 of the certificate will clearly show this. Once the tortoise has been microchipped, you must return the certificate to us for amendment. If there is evidence (such as a statement from your vet) that the physical characteristics of the specimens mean that any method of marking may harm the specimen, we will record this information in box 20 of the certificate. If marking can be safely carried out at a later date, we may issue a certificate containing a special condition.

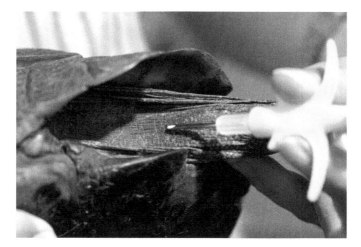

Figure 5.8.1    A microchip implanter pointing to the correct site in the left hind limb for microchip implantation.

Any Annex A tortoise which is being used for commercial gain or being displayed to the public for commercial purposes must be marked. You should remember that the parents of any tortoise being offered for sale will also need to be marked.

*Source*: http://www.defra.gov.uk, accessed September 2012. © Crown Copyright 2012. Contains public sector information licensed under the Open Government Licence v1.0.

From 1st November 2012, Defra have allowed the registration and issued Article 10 certificates for tortoises >60 mm carapace length if marked with a mini-microchip. Tortoises smaller than this still do need to be marked, and this requirement only applies to new applications, and not those already with an Article 10 but not yet marked. Those longer than 10 cm can be marked using either type of microchip.

## Sites

In order to be read correctly, microchips should be placed in the correct site. These recommendations may vary between countries and organisations.

In the United Kingdom, the generally recommended site (from The British Veterinary Zoological Society) is the left hind leg (see Figure 5.8.1), in the gluteal muscles (craniodorsal surface), though the British and Irish Association of Zoos and Aquaria recommends the left shoulder region.

When using the gluteal region, the microchip should be inserted subcutaneously, except in thin-skinned individuals, where it is inserted intramuscularly. In giant tortoises, it may be inserted in the tarsal region of the left hind limb.

However, the gluteal site does have some notable disadvantages. The restraint can be very difficult, with the hind limb hard to grasp and extend in recalcitrant individuals. It is also difficult to disinfect. Subcutaneous implantation can mean that

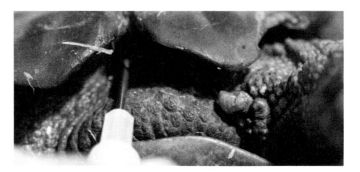

Figure 5.8.2   A microchip being implanted into the midline sub-plastron site.

the chip is easily identified and removed, and is also associated with a higher rate of chip loss post-implantation. The main problem is that there is frequent post-implantation haemorrhage and reaction, especially when the microchip is inserted intramuscularly. Lameness is frequently seen for several days after implantation and owners should be warned accordingly.

Therefore, the midline sub-plastron site is often used instead (see Figure 5.8.2). This site is associated with reduced haemorrhage/reaction and loss of the chip is less common. Restraint is much easier, but skin disinfection can be difficult.

If this site is to be used, the matter of site choice should be discussed with the owner. In smaller species, most scanners will detect a midline chip even if scanned over the left hind leg. However, this may not be the case in larger animals – therefore, if the animal is to be checked/scanned for official purposes (e.g. import/ export), the choice of site may be more important.

More recently, much smaller microchips have become available (e.g. 'Mini-chip'; Micro ID, Scaynes Hill, UK) that are much less traumatic to place and so are strongly recommended, especially in smaller animals.

## Technique

1. Sedation – may be required for hindlimb placement in all animals. It is unlikely to be needed for midline placement. Subcutaneous local anaesthesia is highly recommended for handling and placement in the hind limb, as this is a painful procedure. Midline plastron placement appears less painful and with easier positioning, sedation and local anaesthesia may not be required.
2. Preparation – the implant area should be thoroughly cleaned and then aseptically prepared as for surgery. Skin should be scrubbed with iodine/ chlorhexidine/F10 – a brush can be used for cleaning the leg, and a toothbrush or cotton buds for the midline sub-plastron site.

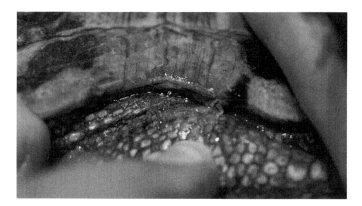

Figure 5.8.3    The midline sub-plastron site post closure with tissue glue.

3.  Insertion – in most animals, the needle can be inserted through the skin. In older thick-skinned animals, a stab incision may be required. The chip implanter should be carefully positioned. Careless insertion can result in damage to:
    a.  the hind limb; blood vessels/nerves – if placed too far proximally/dorsally, there is danger of entry into the lung or kidney.
    b.  the midline – if inserted too far, the chip may be inadvertently placed into the abdomen and, potentially, the bladder.
4.  Closure – in general, tissue glue may be used to close the skin (see Figure 5.8.3). However, a single mattress suture may also be used when placing in the hind limb. This should be removed after 4 weeks.
5.  Post-implantation – the animal should be maintained in a clean environment for a day or two. Semi-aquatic species should be kept out of water for 2 days. The microchip should be rechecked whenever the animal is re-examined.

## Complications

The main complications are infection and/or abscess formation. A good clean technique and reduction of tissue reaction will reduce chances of this.

Other complications are chip loss/migration – adequate placement and skin closure are therefore essential.

# 5.9 Euthanasia

Euthanasia is not always a straightforward procedure in reptiles. Unlike mammals, the slow metabolic rate may mean that death cannot be confirmed until some hours after administration of euthanasia agents.

Therefore, owners should be advised to leave a chelonian at the clinic and collect the following day. If, for any reason, this cannot be done, they should be advised that the animal may move after 'death' and the animal should be sent back with them in a sealed box.

In general, euthanasia is performed by giving intravenous pentobarbitone at a rate of at least 1 ml/500 g. Restraint for intravenous injection can be distressing to some owners, so they may be advised not to be with their pet at this time.

Prior sedation with intramuscular ketamine or alfaxalone may be appropriate and make the task easier.

For small animals, intracardiac injection may be appropriate; however, prior sedation must always be given (see Figure 5.9.1).

See Chapter 5.1.

Intracoelomic injection is not advised unless the other routes are unachievable, as intracoelomic injection may be painful and uptake can be very variable.

Once the animal is completely unconscious, death may be completed by:

- waiting
- freezing
- brain pithing
- decapitation

## Determination of death

This is a common request after very debilitated tortoises are presented by owners, post-euthanasia and during anaesthetic crises.

Some cases are obvious, with extensive necrosis/rigor mortis. Others are less so and the following tests may be performed:

1. Absence of all pain/withdrawal/blink reflexes.

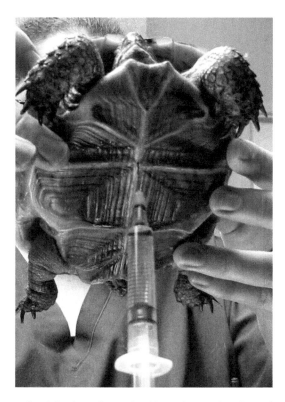

Figure 5.9.1   Intracardiac injection of pentobarbitone in a sedated tortoise. Note the location of the heart, marked by the intersection of scutes. Note too that the tortoise must not be turned upside down or the heart will 'flop' away from this site.

2.  ECG – however, weak signals may be undetectable using standard small-animal equipment. Conversely, an ECG signal may be detected for up to 24 hours following apparent death by euthanasia – this may represent ventricular pacing.
3.  8 MHz Doppler – detection of an obvious heart beat. Place the probe between the extended neck and front leg (see Chapter 6). The heart rate is probably very slow, so the probe should be left in each position for several minutes and repositioned several times. This device is commonly found in small-animal practices, where it is used for indirect blood pressure assessment in cats.
4.  Ultrasound – use the same site as for 8 MHz Doppler. This may be deemed more sensitive, as heart movement may be easier to detect visually rather than audibly. As in technique 3 above, the heart should be observed over several minutes before death is declared.

# 6 General Anaesthesia

Anaesthesia is now a common procedure in chelonian medicine, to allow diagnostic procedures or for surgery. It may be a brief anaesthetic – for example, to facilitate a clinical examination – or prolonged, for a complicated surgical operation. With improved understanding of reptilian physiology the safety of anaesthesia in reptile species has evolved significantly over recent years.

A satisfactory outcome for the patient relies on the anaesthetist having the necessary knowledge and practical skills and being able to effectively integrate this knowledge with planning the procedure, situation awareness, team-working, communication and decision-making in the operating theatre environment.

The decision to anaesthetise must be based on a thorough examination and history-taking and a rational diagnostic/treatment plan. The potential risks versus the benefits need to be evaluated and discussed with the owner.

## Assessment before general anaesthesia

### History

The history should include signalment, environment, diet, presenting signs and any previous medical history.

### Clinical examination

A thorough clinical examination, including an assessment of the body, is essential. It is important to remember that chelonian species are very stoical, hiding signs of illness, and can be very ill by the time the owner notices that there is a problem.

### Diagnostic testing

Diagnostic testing prior to anaesthesia depends on the patient and on the presenting clinical signs, the underlying disease and the history of individual and/ or group and/or the geographical location. The initial results may indicate that

*Essentials of Tortoise Medicine and Surgery*, First Edition. John Chitty and Aidan Raftery.
© 2013 John Chitty and Aidan Raftery. Published 2013 by John Wiley & Sons, Ltd.

further diagnostic testing is required. The minimum recommended database before general anaesthesia is as follows:

- uric acid
- urea
- glucose
- PCV
- blood smear evaluation
- sodium
- potassium
- ionised calcium if reproductive or any suspicion of a metabolic bone disorder

## Preparation, equipment and skills needed

- The anaesthetic must be monitored by an assistant who has the appropriate training and experience. The anaesthetist should not be distracted by having to procure needed equipment and should not have to assist with the surgery/procedure.
- Draw up a crash plan and ensure that all relevant staff are conversant with their part. Intubate if not already intubated. Commence positive-pressure ventilation, using 100% oxygen at a rate of 6–10 breaths per minute. In cases of cardiac arrest, give adrenaline/epinephrine 0.1 mg/kg intravenously or intra-osseously, or double this dose down the endotracheal tube.
- Chelonians can be resuscitated after long periods of respiratory arrest. They have also been revived after periods of apparent cardiac arrest. If revived, they are unlikely to have any ischemia- or reperfusion-related damage.
- All the equipment that might be needed for the procedure should be prepared in advance and be close at hand.
- Plan for the post-anaesthetic care in addition to that associated with the surgery; for example, provide nutritional support and appropriate analgesia, and have a suitable recovery area ready.

## Preparation of the patient

- In many cases, initiating treatment before a general anaesthetic may reduce the anaesthetic risk and in some cases make the procedure unnecessary.
- It is vital that the patient is stable before anaesthesia is induced.
- Supportive care is essential:
  - fluid therapy
  - effective analgesia
  - thermal support
  - nutritional support

A balanced analgesia plan has a big impact on recovery, and this starts before or just after the induction of anaesthesia.

## Induction

A mask or anaesthetic chamber induction is not possible, as Chelonia can breath-hold for very long periods. Induction is by either intravenous or intramuscular injection.

## Intubation

- This can be difficult due to poor visibility of the glottis, especially in smaller individuals.
- The glottis is positioned behind the tongue.
- Pathological changes in the oral cavity make intubation even more difficult.
- Place a finger in the intramandibular area and push upwards: this brings the glottis forward, making intubation easier.
- Wait for the glottis to open as the animal breathes, and slip in the tube approximately 2–3 cm.
- The protruding end of the endotracheal tube is then taped to a rigid support that is attached to the patient's head and to the ventilator, ensuring that they all move as one. Also, keep the head and neck straight to avoid any trauma that the tip of the tube may cause on the endothelial lining of the trachea.
- Endotracheal tubes have to be improvised for the smaller patients. Intravenous over-the-needle catheters can be used.
- The smallest tubes are much more prone to obstruction with mucus, so this must be monitored closely.
- Do not place too far down as in some species the trachea divides quickly, so that there is a risk of intubation of only one bronchus. Cole-pattern endotracheal tubes are used by some, as the wider top section of these tubes prevents deep placement of the tube and also helps seal the glottis for ventilation.

## Maintenance

Isoflurane or sevoflurane gaseous inhalation agents are commonly used to maintain general anaesthesia.

A ventilator is important, especially in longer procedures. The peak airway pressure should be set at 12–15 cm $H_2O$ with a respiratory rate of 4–8 breaths per minute. Manual ventilation can be used; however, care is needed as damage can be caused by overinflation.

## Positioning

- Positioning is dictated by the procedure; however, individuals with pneumonia will be compromised by placing them in dorsal recumbency.
- The position must be stable to stop movement during surgery.

# Recovery

- Recovery can be slow, especially from longer procedures and in compromised individuals. The recovery rate also depends on the anaesthetic regime.

- Maintain on the ventilator until obviously breathing on their own or conscious enough and trying to move. As in other reptiles, respiration in chelonians is stimulated by high $CO_2$ and low $O_2$ levels. Recovery can sometimes be very slow, especially in debilitated individuals. Causing hypoxia and hypercapnia in an attempt to stimulate respiration is risky. It is safer to only extubate when oral and pharyngeal reflexes have returned, which usually coincides with the first signs of limb and jaw movement.
- It is critical to monitor core body temperature, especially when recovery is prolonged.
- Use reversal agents where possible.

## Emergencies

Resuscitation techniques should be practiced in advance and there should always be a simple crash box present with quick-reference dose charts for the doses of emergency drugs. There is a much longer window after respiratory arrest when resuscitation is possible. Chelonians can also be recovered from apparent cardiac arrest more readily than mammalian or avian species.

### Respiratory arrest

- Stop anaesthetic administration and check the heart rate.
- Place an endotracheal tube if not already present.
- Position in ventral recumbency.
- Start positive-pressure ventilation, using 100% oxygen at a rate of 6–10 breaths per minute.
- Monitor the heart rate.

### Cardiac arrest

- Give adrenaline/epinephrine 0.1 mg/kg intravenously or intra-osseously, or double this dose down the endotracheal tube.
- There will be concurrent respiratory arrest, which needs treating as above.

## Monitoring

- Doppler flow detector – a probe is placed over a peripheral artery, allowing the heart rate to be monitored by an audible signal. Usually, the carotid artery is used. This is the most useful piece of monitoring equipment in Chelonia.
- The temperature should be maintained within the preferred optimum temperature range. Hypothermia is a major concern, especially in smaller patients, and is often the cause of prolonged recoveries. A temperature probe either placed in the oesophagus or cloaca will allow the necessary adjustments to be made in time. Supplemental heat can be provided by a combination of heated operating tables, forced-air warming blankets or circulation water blankets.

- Electrocardiography is useful for detecting cardiac arrhythmias. Early bradycardia and st segment depression are often the first signs of anaesthetic overdose. However, it is important to remember that the electrocardiogram may be normal in the face of severe cardiopulmonary compromise.
- The pulse oximeter is less useful due to its reduced accuracy in chelonian patients: probes that can be placed into the cloaca or oesophagus are the most reliable. It is best used to monitor trends.

## Anaesthetic protocols

Many different anaesthetic protocols have been published for chelonians. A protocol should ideally result in a smooth induction with a rapid recovery. Agents that can be reversed or are rapidly cleared from the body are preferred. The dose can vary significantly depending on the condition of the patient, so doses will need to be adjusted for debilitated animals. It is safer for the clinician and the nursing staff to be very familiar with one or two protocols.

1. Alfaxalone 4–9 mg/kg intravenously, with higher doses for smaller individuals and the lower end of the dose rate needed for the giant tortoises. This gives approximately 20 minutes of surgical anaesthesia and can be topped up with repeat doses as necessary. Alternatively, they can be intubated and maintained under anaesthesia with isoflurane or sevoflurane inhalation anaesthesia.
2. Propofol at 4–10 mg/kg intravenously, then intubate for ventilation. Anaesthesia is usually maintained with isoflurane or sevoflurane inhalation anaesthesia.
3. Midazolam 0.2 mg/kg and hydromorphone 0.1 mg/kg by intramuscular injection as a premed, then induce with propofol 3–4 mg/kg intravenously. Reverse with flumazenil 0.008 mg/kg.
4. Midazolam 1 mg/kg and medetomidine 0.1 mg/kg (or dexmedetomidine 0.065 mg/kg) and ketamine 2.5–5 mg/kg by intramuscular injection. Analgesia can be enhanced by adding in morphine 1.5 mg/kg or hydromorphone 0.1 mg/kg, by intramuscular injection as a premed. Afterwards, reverse with 0.008 mg/kg flumazenil IV and 0.5 mg/kg atipamezole intramuscularly.
5. Ketamine 1 mg/kg and midazolam 0.2 mg/kg, and medetomidine 0.01 mg/kg IM. Then, if necessary, give propofol at 2 mg/kg intravenously. Afterwards, reverse with flumazenil 0.008 mg/kg IV and atipamezole 0.05 mg/kg IM.
6. Hydromorphone 0.05 mg/kg and midazolam 0.2 mg/kg IM. Reverse the midazolam with flumazenil at 0.008 mg/kg.

## Pain management

- Morphine has been demonstrated to have analgesic properties in reptiles.
- Hydromorphone is a more potent analgesic than morphine and uses the same receptor sites.
- Buprenorphine and butorphanol have not been shown to have analgesic properties in reptiles.

- Non-steroidal anti-inflammatory drugs are usually used in conjunction with opiates.
- Local analgesia should be provided with an incisional block: lignocaine mixed with bupivicaine diluted for smaller individuals. The total dose is dictated by the surgical site, but keep the total dose below 2 mg/kg for each drug.
- Tramadol orally at 10 mg/kg can be given every 48 hours.

# 7 Imaging

## 7.1 Radiography

High-resolution capability is required to provide diagnostic radiographs from the smallest to the very large animal. High-resolution film screen systems – for example, mammography film/screen systems – will provide good diagnostic radiographs; however, exposure settings and the processing have a big impact on the quality of the films. Digital systems, with their enhanced processing power, are much more tolerant of exposure settings and it is easier to consistently produce diagnostic images from a range of patient sizes.

Radiology in chelonians is most useful for the evaluation of the skeletal system, lungs, the urinary tract, the reproductive tract and the gastrointestinal tract. Evaluation of other soft tissue structures is compromised by the presence of the shell (refer to Figures 1.4.3 and 1.4.4 for normal organ positions).

### Views

There are three views that are commonly taken. Ideally, the animal should be in ventral recumbency for all views, with a horizontal beam required for the lateral and craniocaudal views. If the animal is positioned for these views so that a vertical beam can be used, displacement of viscus will affect interpretation, especially of the lung fields:

- Dorsoventral view – this is the best view to evaluate the urinary tract, the reproductive tract, the gastrointestinal tract and the skeletal system. The animal is positioned in ventral recumbency directly on the plate, with the head and four limbs extended if possible.
- Lateral view – the animal is positioned on a pedestal so that the legs have no purchase. The X-ray machine is positioned perpendicular to the animal, centred

on the bridge so as to produce a horizontal beam. The plate should be touching the animal and perpendicular to the X-ray beam. This view provides the best views of the viscera and the vertebrae. On average, the lung fields should occupy approximately the dorsal 50% of the coelomic cavity and the viscera the ventral 50% (see Figure 7.1.1).

- Craniocaudal or skyline view – for this view, a horizontal X-ray beam is projected in a craniocaudal direction. The animal has to be slightly elevated on a pedestal so that the legs are hanging down. This position provides a view of each lung (see Figure 7.1.2).

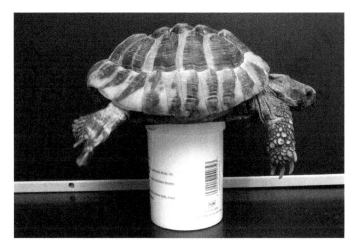

Figure 7.1.1    Positioning for the lateral view.

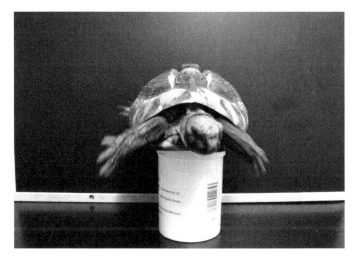

Figure 7.1.2    Positioning for the craniocaudal view.

## Contrast views

Barium sulphate is the most frequently used contrast material. It is used to image the gastrointestinal tract and to give information on gastrointestinal motility:

- Dose 10 ml per kilogram body weight.
- Barium sulphate has a slow gut transit time, which can amount to days. More dilute concentrations will have more rapid transit times (see Figures 7.1.3 and 7.1.4).
- Iodinated non-ionic contrast media – for example, iohexol – have faster gut transit times. Iohexol is commonly used at the same dose rate. Iohexol is indicated if a gastrointestinal perforation is suspected.
- Warm the contrast material to body temperature.
- Administer by stomach tube.
- Transit through the entire gastrointestinal tract can take several days.
- Do not allow the animal to become dehydrated after administering barium sulphate.

Contrast material occasionally needs to be used in the bladder to evaluate whether an object seen radiographically is in the bladder.

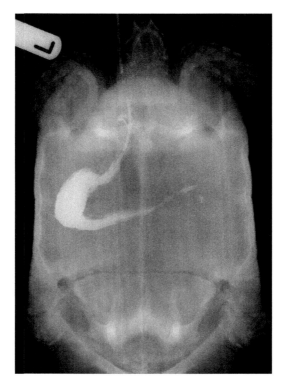

Figure 7.1.3    Barium administration via an oesophageal feeding tube: the position of the stomach.

- Eggs can sometimes be found in the urinary bladder. They often have a thickened rough shell appearance due to the accumulation of urate deposits.
- Urinary calculi may be difficult to differentiate from pebbles or other material in the gastrointestinal tract.
- The chelonian bladder is very large when full and extends far forward.
- Iodinated non-ionic contrast media – for example, iohexol – can be used at 10–20 ml/kg.
- Air can be added to provide a double contrast, in which case reduce the positive contrast material to approximately 5 ml/kg.
- Air should be removed from the bladder afterwards.
- Cystoscopy facilitates biopsy of soft tissue masses in the bladder.
- Ultrasound can provide complementary information.

## Common findings and interpretation

### Gastrointestinal system

- Small pebbles and sand are a common normal finding. They often remain in the dilated portion of the transverse colon for prolonged periods. This is on the left side, but may sometimes extend across towards the right side (see Figure 38.1).
- Obstructions may not be obvious on a plain radiograph unless they are radio-opaque material.

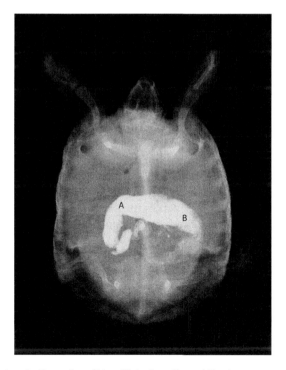

Figure 7.1.4   Barium in the colon: (A) a dilated portion of the transverse colon; (B) the proximal colon.

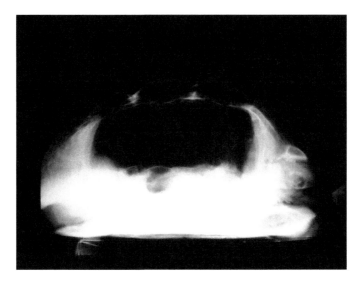

Figure 7.1.5    A radiograph of a normal lung: the lateral view.

- Contrast studies are needed to confirm obstructions.
- Normally, there will be little gas present. Excess gas is associated with ileus. The cause has to be identified.

## Musculoskeletal system

- Evaluate bone density (see Chapter 17).
- Careful positioning will make visualisation of limb fractures easier. If the limbs are retracted, then the shell can hide fractures or bone pathology. Additionally, some fractures will be reduced when the limbs are withdrawn, so the diagnosis will be missed.
- In the absence of a normal image, compare the right and left sides.
- Arthritis can sometimes be diagnosed radiographically.
- Radiolucent areas are usually significant.
- Mineralisation of soft tissues such as muscle is sometimes seen.
- Chronically inflamed areas can become mineralised.

## Respiratory system

See Figures 7.1.5 and 7.1.6.

- Mild (and sometimes severe) disease of the lower respiratory tract usually does not produce changes on radiographs.
- Evaluate if unilateral or bilateral (see Figure 7.1.7).
- Focal lesions can be localised for access via a carapace osteotomy.

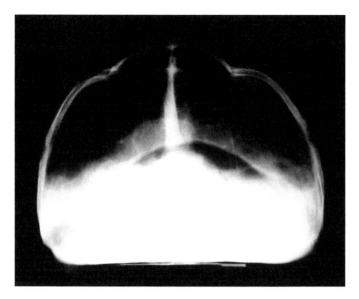

Figure 7.1.6   A radiograph of a normal lung: the craniocaudal view.

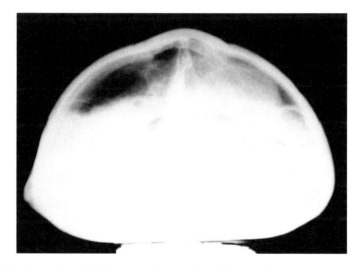

Figure 7.1.7   A craniocaudal view revealing a unilateral lung lesion.

## Urinary system

- The bladder has a very large capacity.
- Calculi are commonly found. Small calculi are usually asymptomatic.
- Calculi can also be seen in the cloaca. Some of these are radiolucent.
- Contrast studies, ultrasound and cystoscopy will help further evaluate the urinary system. See above for contrast doses.

- Pebbles in the gastrointestinal system can be confused with urinary calculi. Contrast studies help here.

## Genital system

- Eggs should be seen on the radiograph, with dystocia.
- Evaluate the number and shape of eggs.
- Thickened shells may indicate that they have been there for a long time.
- Occasionally, eggs can be found in the urinary bladder. Contrast studies or ultrasound may be needed to clarify their position.
- Follicles are not seen on radiographs; ultrasound is indicated if they are suspected
- Broken eggs usually require a coelotomy.
- Abnormal masses or calculi can cause dystocia.

# 7.2  Ultrasound

Diagnostic ultrasound is a very useful technique in chelonian medicine for imaging soft tissue structures:

- It is non-invasive.
- Only some individuals will need sedation, so that the imaging windows can be accessed.
- The usefulness is limited by the skill of the operator and his/her knowledge of the normal anatomy of the species.
- The bony shell of chelonians is a barrier to ultrasound.

High-resolution ultrasonography significantly improves the diagnostic capabilities, given the limitations of the chelonian patient. Except for the giant chelonians, a 7.5 mHz transducer with a small footprint is recommended. In the giant chelonians, a 5 mHz transducer is used.

## Sonic windows

- The cervicobrachial window is used to image the heart, major blood vessels and thyroid. The liver and gall bladder lie caudal to the heart and can also be visualised via this window (see Figure 7.2.1).
- The pre-femoral window provides ultrasound access to the reproductive tract and bladder. Depending on the anatomy of the pre-femoral fossa, the degree of visualisation of the kidneys and liver will vary with the species. It is often difficult to view the gastrointestinal tract due to the presence of gas. If there is gas affecting the view, then try from the opposite side (see Figure 7.2.2).
- Soft-shelled turtles and pancake tortoises can often be scanned through the plastron due to the nature of their shell. Water is an effective stand-off, so the ultrasound can be performed while they are held in the water.
- The eye, depending on size and on the equipment used, can be scanned to visualise ocular and retrobulbar soft tissue structures.

The transducer can be placed directly on the skin after the liberal application of ultrasound transmission gel or a stand-off can be used; or, alternatively, the area of the sonic window can be submerged in water and the transducer placed in the water and directed towards the available window.

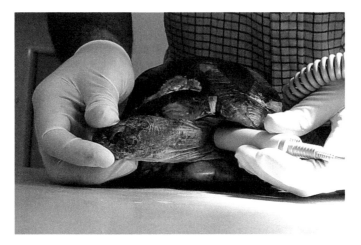

Figure 7.2.1    Ultrasound through the cervicobrachial sonic window.
*Source*: McArthur, S., Wilkinson, R. and Meyer, J. (eds) (2004) *Medicine and Surgery of Tortoises and Turtles*. Reproduced with permission of John Wiley & Sons, Ltd.

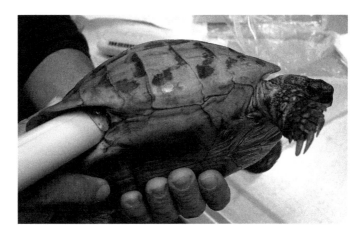

Figure 7.2.2    Ultrasound through the pre-femoral sonic window.

## The reproductive tract

Evaluation of the reproductive tract is the most common use of ultrasound in chelonians.

- Ovaries can be followed through the reproductive cycle.
- Abnormalities such as pre-ovulatory ova stasis and dystocia can be diagnosed.
- Treatment is influenced by the detail of the findings – for example, whether a dystocia case is obstructive or non-obstructive.
- Pre-ovulatory ova stasis requires a series of ultrasounds (sonograms) to document that there is stasis.

## The bladder

If full, the bladder can be imaged and the presence of calculi or eggs identified.

## The liver

The liver can be evaluated for:

- size and shape
- irregularities of the parenchyma, such as:
  - cystic structures
  - abscesses
  - neoplasia
- Venous congestion, where the differentials would include:
  - hepatic disease
  - cardiac disease
- The gall bladder should be identified in the dorsal aspect of the right lobe.

## The heart

The three-chambered heart and major vessels are identified through the cervico-brachial window. Measurements normally taken in mammalian sonography are unreliable in chelonians due to the irregularity of their myocardium. Irregularities that can be identified include:

- cardiomegaly
- pericardial fluid
- cardiac masses
- endocarditis

## The gastrointestinal tract

The pre-femoral window gives best access to the gastrointestinal tract. It can be evaluated for:

- soft tissue masses
- foreign bodies
- atonic dilated loops of bowel
- excess gas, which will compromise its evaluation

## The kidneys

Chelonian kidneys are not always easy to image due to the angle of the pre-femoral window and their anatomical position. When imaged, they should appear triangular in shape.

# 7.3 Endoscopy and Biopsy

## Equipment needed

- Endoscopes ranging in size from 1 mm to 4 mm in diameter, depending on the anatomical site and the size of the patient. Rigid endoscopes are more commonly used, but flexible endoscopes can be used in the gastrointestinal tract and the respiratory tract. For narrow tubular organs, a 0 degree angle is preferred. In body spaces, a 30 degree angle is most often used, as it gives a wider angle of view as it is rotated around.
- Light source.
- Sheath – this is to protect the endoscope and will usually have channels for passing instruments, insufflation gas and fluids for irrigation.
- Trochar.
- Gas insufflator – this may be stand-alone or combined with the light source. Carbon dioxide is the preferred gas due to the reduced risk of a gaseous embolism.
- Endoscope camera – although it is possible to use the scope looking directly through the eyepiece, use of a camera with the procedure viewed on a screen is easier once familiar with the technique, and in some situations allows two operators, which facilitates more complex procedures.
- Instruments:

  - biopsy forceps
  - scissors
  - grasping forceps
  - needles for aspiration and injection

*Extra items*

Any additional items that may be needed during the procedure should be prepared in advance: materials for the collection of diagnostic samples – for example, containers for histopathology, swabs with transport material, microscope slides for cytology or any specialised media/containers that may be required.

## Areas

### *Coelioscopy*

*Indications*
- Investigation of disease involving structures in the coelomic cavity.
- Samples can be collected for cytology, histology, microbial cultures and other microbial tests.
- Intra-lesion treatment of localised lesions is occasionally possible.

*Position*
- The animal is best positioned in lateral recumbency.
- It will need to be supported in this position.
- The choice of which side is dependent on whether lesions were detected on radiography or ultrasound.
- The hind leg is extended to expose the pre-femoral fossa and secured in position.
- Endoscopically assisted surgical procedures may require the animal to be in dorsal recumbency.

*Preparation*
- General anaesthetic is required.
- The skin needs to be prepared as if for surgery and surgically draped.
- All required equipment and materials must be prepared and ready for use before anaesthesia is induced.
- Familiarity with normal anatomy is essential.

*Approach*
- A small stab incision is made centrally in the pre-femoral fossa.
- Larger incisions will be necessary if this is to be an endoscopically assisted surgery.
- The subcutaneous tissues are separated to the aponeurosis of the transverse and oblique abdominal muscles.
- The aponeurosis is bluntly dissected into the coelomic cavity.
- Insufflication of the coelom will be necessary to achieve good visibility. Carbon dioxide insufflication carries a much reduced risk of a gaseous embolism.
- Insufflication pressures should be between 3 and 5 mmHg.
- Gas should be removed from the coelum after the procedure.
- On completion, the aponeurosis and the skin are sutured separately.
- The skin can be closed with sutures or skin staples.
- Aquatic species should be dry docked for 24 hours.

*Complications*
- Most complications are associated with an incorrect approach.
- The approach can deviate into the femoral musculature.
- The lung space may be entered.
- If the peritoneal membrane is separated but not penetrated, there will not be a clear view and diagnostic samples cannot be collected.
- If at the wrong angle, the approach may end up tunnelling through soft tissues.
- Haemorrhage can obscure the view.

- Cloudy fluid in the coelomic cavity can obscure the view.
- Hepatomegaly can result in the liver being penetrated during a blunt approach.
- Gas left in the coelum may alter the buoyancy in aquatic and semi-aquatic species. In humans, gas left inside the coelum is a major cause of post-procedure pain.
- Air embolism can occur from the insufflication gas, especially if the pressure was too high.

## External nares

### Indications
- Unilateral discharge.
- Discharge from the choana.
- Distortion of the maxillary/nasal bones.
- Non-responsive bilateral nasal discharge.

### Position
- The animal should be in ventral recumbency.

### Preparation.
- General anaesthetic – or, at a minimum, sedation – is required.
- A rigid scope that will fit through the external nares is chosen.

### Approach
- Both external nares should be examined.
- Flushing may be required if there is discharge present.
- Examine the choana from an intra-oral approach. A scope with a 30 degree angle field of view will be needed here.

### Complications
- Trauma, especially if the animal moves.
- Damage to the endoscopes.
- Haemorrhage.

## Lower respiratory tract tracheal approach

### Indications
- Discharge from the glottis.
- Respiratory sounds.
- Inflammation; swelling of the glottis.
- Tracheal lesion identified on clinical examination or diagnostic imaging.

### Position
- The animal is placed in ventral recumbency.
- A 20 degree angled slope up towards the head will help reduce the risk of aspiration.

### Preparation
- A 0 degree rigid scope is preferred.
- Scopes with angled views are more likely to cause trauma to the lining of the trachea on introduction.
- A general anaesthetic is essential.

*Approach*
- The oropharynx and the glottis should be examined.
- Wait for inspiration.
- The scope is passed through the glottis.

*Complications*
- Iatrogenic trauma to the lining of the trachea.
- Penetration of the trachea at the bifurcation or lower.

## Lower respiratory tract carapace approach

*Indications*
- Focal lung lesion, where the position is already identified by diagnostic imaging.
- Sampling of the lesion.
- Complete removal can occasionally be accomplished.
- Intra-lesion drug delivery.

*Position*
- The animal should be positioned in ventral recumbency.

*Preparation*
- A general anaesthetic is required, as this is an osteotomy.
- The surgical site must be aseptically prepared. Any grooves or folds in the surgical area will need to be thoroughly cleaned with a small scrubbing brush or toothbrush.
- The animal needs to be intubated and ideally placed on a ventilator so that the lung pressure can be monitored.

*Approach*
- An osteotomy is created in the carapace over the lesion.
- Just slightly larger than the endoscope.
- The pleuroperitoneal membrane is penetrated with a trocar and the sheath. Ideally, try to maintain a tight seal.
- The trocar is withdrawn and the endoscope is advanced through the sheath, allowing visualisation.
- The opening can be sealed permanently. Alternatively, a catheter can be placed in the lungs, with an injection cap. This is then temporarily sealed in place with sterile bone wax. This allows repeat access.

*Complications*
- Inflammation at the entry site may cause swelling and exudates, which may further compromise respiration.
- If entry through the pleuroperitoneal membrane was difficult, a space may have been created between the carapace and the pleuroperitonal membrane where air can accumulate and reduce the space for expansion of the lungs.
- Post-operative infection.
- Dissemination of an initially localised infection.

## Lower respiratory tract pre-femoral approach

### Indications
- Diffuse lung disease, where a tracheal/lung wash has been non-diagnostic.

### Position
- Lateral recumbency, with the affected side uppermost.
- The hind limb is taped back to expose the pre-femoral fossa.

### Preparation
- The skin and surrounding areas of carapace and plastron are surgically prepared.
- Burring back the horn of the edge of the plastron will improve access. Trans-illuminate so as not to expose bone.
- A general anaesthetic is required.
- The animal needs to be intubated and ideally placed on a ventilator so that the lung pressure can be monitored.

### Approach
- A linear craniocaudal incision is made in the skin of the pre-femoral fossa.
- The incision should be in the craniodorsal quadrant of the pre-femoral fossa.
- Inflation of the lungs will aid the placement of stay sutures in the lung.
- A stab incision allows entry of the endoscope.

### Complications
- Pneumocoelum will occur if the lung incision is not closed.
- Infected exudates may leak into coelom, causing a coelomitis.
- Post-operative infection.

## Gastrointestinal tract

### Indications
- Retrieval of foreign bodies.
- Biopsy of lesions.
- Investigation of gastrointestinal disease.

### Position
- Ventral recumbency, although some operators prefer dorsal recumbency.
- The head is extended.
- An angled approach, with the head higher than the vent, will reduce the risk of aspiration.

### Preparation
- Ideally, the animal should be fasted for a period to reduce the stomach contents. Carnivorous species should be fasted for approximately 3 days and herbivorous species for 4–5 days.
- A general anaesthetic is required.
- The trachea should be intubated.

### Approach
- A flexible or rigid endoscope is introduced through the oral cavity.

- Care must be taken not to damage the thin-walled oesophagus. This can most readily happen with the rigid endoscopes that have an angled view.
- Gas insufflation or body-temperature saline can be used to dilate the oesophagus for entry.
- Insufflation is necessary to visualise the tract.

*Complications*
- Pain from a distended bowel, caused by too much insufflation gas.
- Trauma to the lining of the gut by the endoscope.
- The presence of fluids or ingesta, obscuring visibility.

## Urinary bladder (Cystoscopy)

*Indications*
- Investigation of haematuria or other bladder-related symptom.
- Removal of eggs or bladder stones.

*Position*
- Ventral recumbency.
- Sloping at a 30 degree angle, head down with the vent at the edge of the table.

*Preparation*
- A general anaesthetic is essential.
- Body-temperature saline must be ready to infuse into the cloaca and bladder, to allow good visualisation.

*Approach*
- The scope is introduced into the cloaca.
- The entrance into the bladder is in the floor of the urodeum.
- The urethra is very short.
- The bladder is thin walled and usually bilobed.

*Complications*
- Chronic urolithiasis can make the bladder wall weaker and more prone to rupture.
- Trauma on introduction of the endoscope to the cloacal tissues, urethra and the bladder.

## Cloacoscopy

*Indications*
- Masses seen on radiography or ultrasound may be visualised and sampled if necessary.
- Eggs and uroliths in the cloaca may be manipulated through the vent. Eggs are punctured and a Foley catheter (filled with frozen water to make it more rigid for ease of placement) is placed in the hole, inflated to fill the egg and then withdrawn. Bladder eggs are removed in the same way. Uroliths are snared with endoscopic baskets and then removed.
- The cloaca can be examined.
- The colon can be entered and sampled.

- The oviduct opening can be visualised. Eggs in the opening or distal oviduct may be imploded.
- Discharges from urethra or oviduct can be observed and sampled if necessary.
- The phallus and the clitoris can be examined.
- Prolapsed tissue may be identified.
- Small masses can be removed.

*Position*
- The animal is positioned in ventral recumbency, with the operator seated behind. If the endoscope is not attached to a camera, the surgeon will need to have the animal at eye level.
- Positioning on a slanting surface, head down, will facilitate retention of fluid in the cloaca, giving better visualisation.

*Preparation*
- A general anaesthetic may be needed, depending on the pathology present and the condition of the patient.
- Debilitated patients will not need sedation/general anaesthetic.
- Urates and faecal material may need to be flushed out.
- Colonoscopy requires flushing faecal material from the colon.

*Approach*
- The cloaca is approached through the vent.
- The margins between the different sections of the cloaca are often indistinct
- Body-temperature saline or lubricant gel can be infused in to the cloaca to improve visualisation.
- The vent has to be held shut around the scope to keep the cloaca distended.

*Complications*
- Cloacal or oviduct trauma during attempts to puncture eggs or break down uroliths for removal.
- Haemorrhage, especially from friable or devitalised tissues.
- Small haemorrhages will obscure the view.

# 7.4 Advanced Imaging Techniques

Computed tomography (CT) and magnetic resonance imaging (MRI) are still rarely performed in Chelonia, even though they are becoming more accessible to veterinarians, and can provide valuable information.

The principal reason is that of cost and because these imaging modalities are rarely held by clinicians familiar with Chelonia.

## Computed tomography

Indications for CT are as follows:

- particularly appropriate for examination of the skeletal system, including the shell
- spinal injury, including narrowing of the spinal canal
- observation and measurement of soft tissue densities in the respiratory system
- internal organs – for example, the liver and ovaries – and eggs can be assessed and measured
- gastrointestinal foreign bodies

Slice thicknesses of 1–2 mm should be used when scanning and CT data can be interpreted using the same programmes as for mammals.

CT scans generally take less time than MRI.

Movement artefacts should be reduced by sedating or anaesthetising the animal. In conscious animals, the legs may be taped inside the shell.

### Magnetic resonance imaging

As this takes longer than CT, movement artefact is more easily achieved. Therefore animals will require sedation/anaesthesia for MRI examination.

Slice thicknesses of 2–6 mm are used, with a field of view between 150 and 190 mm.

MRI can provide fine detail on all internal soft tissues and may be indicated to assess:

- organomegaly
- space-occupying lesions

- assessment of ovary and eggs
- gastrointestinal foreign bodies
- respiratory disease – especially in assessing pneumonia

## Further reading

Krautwald-Junghanns, M.-E., Pees, M., Reese, S. & Tully, T. (2011) *Diagnostic Imaging of Exotic Pets*. Schlutersche, Hannover, Germany. This title provides an excellent basic guide to these imaging modalities in Chelonia.

# 8    Surgery

## 8.1    Surgery Needs and Equipment

There are specialist instrument requirements for operating on chelonians. However, these are in addition to the routine instruments and equipment used in surgery on other species.

### Coeliotomy requirements

- A cutting disc that dissipates heat rapidly, for the surgical entry.
- A drill that takes the cutting disc.
- Goggles for protection of the surgical team during the use of the cutting disc.
- Quick-setting resin for sealing the surgical entry site.

### Anaesthetic equipment

- Endotracheal tubes, 1–4 mm uncuffed.
- A ventilator ideally, or at a minimum an ambu bag.
- A Doppler pencil or flat probe – the 8 MHz frequency is recommended.
- A temperature probe to monitor the core temperature.

Staff should be trained in anaesthetic monitoring and emergency procedures.

### Critical care and surgical recovery

- A critical care unit or an improvised environment to be used as a recovery area, or for stabilisation of critical patients. The temperature and humidity should be controllable.

*Essentials of Tortoise Medicine and Surgery*, First Edition. John Chitty and Aidan Raftery.
© 2013 John Chitty and Aidan Raftery. Published 2013 by John Wiley & Sons, Ltd.

- Vivariums already set up so that animals can be immediately placed in their preferred optimum temperature zone.
- Syringe drivers and/or infusion pumps.

## Surgery

Working deep in the coelomic cavity imposes certain limitations, which can be reduced by using the correct equipment.

- Vascular clips.
- Long-handled instruments.
- Cotton tips.
- Bulldog surgical clamps or equivalent are invaluable.
- Clear plastic adhesive drapes allow easier monitoring and retention of heat, which is especially important in the smaller patients.
- Use suture material that elicits a minimal reaction. Polydioxanone (PDS), Polyglyconate (Maxon), Glycomer 631 (Biosyn), Polyglecaprone 25 (Monocryl) and Polyglytone 6211 (Caprosyn) are examples of suture materials that produce minimum inflammation and minimum tissue drag.

## Endoscopy system

An invaluable diagnostic tool in chelonian medicine.

- Needle scope (1.2 mm) with a 0 degree angle.
- A 1.9–2.7 mm scope with a 0 or 30 degree angle. It should have a sheath with an instrument channel through which biopsy forceps and scissors can fit.

## Radiosurgery

Very useful, but not essential. Monopolar and bipolar are both useful, especially for the delicate surgery needed on the smaller patients.

## Radiology

The following are essential:

- Horizontal beam exposure capability is especially important to image the lungs.
- Digital radiography has greatly increased the value of radiographs, especially in the smaller patients, due to its ability to improve image quality by reducing noise, removing technical artefacts and optimising contrast. Additionally, image manipulation enables proper evaluation of bone and soft tissue on the same plate without two exposures.

## Dremel

A dremel (or similar) with grinding stones for beaks and nails.

## Tools for opening beak and oral examinations

Dental instruments are very useful in this respect. They are also useful for probing abscesses, wounds and so on.

# 8.2 Haemostasis

Haemostasis is as important in reptiles as in other animals. Excessive blood loss will lead to circulatory shock and death. In healthy individuals, a blood loss of 1% of body weight is safe. With higher blood losses, clinical signs will become more evident.

The following factors affect blood coagulation:

- hepatopathy
- hibernation
- septicaemia
- anti-coagulant drug toxicity

Chronic anaemia will lead to a reduction in thrombocyte numbers, as they are recruited to become erythrocytes.

During surgery, good haemostasis is essential, especially when in the coelomic cavity. Sutures can be difficult to place deep in the cavity. Tying the knot outside the coelomic cavity and tightening it up with a knot pusher results in good ligatures and minimal tissue damage on placement. Alternatively, there are various makes of vascular clips available, with applicators of different lengths and shapes. Radiosurgery, $CO_2$ and diode lasers allow relatively bloodless dissection. Smaller blood vessels are sealed.

Traumatic wounds, if bleeding, can have the haemorrhage controlled by pressure using a sterile surgical swab, or in an emergency with clean cotton or paper towelling by the owner, prior to veterinary emergency treatment. As in mammalian medicine, major blood vessels may need to be ligated.

Chelonians, especially the terrestrial species, cope better with blood loss than mammals; however, treatment is required in serious acute blood loss. There are no real guidelines on when a blood transfusion or oxyglobin will be required. The decision is best based on the clinical condition of the animal, as the symptoms depend on the rapidity of the blood loss. Oxyglobin can be used at 5 ml/kg intravenously or intraosseously as a bolus. Blood transfusions can be harvested from disease-free animals of the same species at 1% of body weight, and then given intravenously or intraosseously slowly as a bolus.

# 8.3    Surgical Techniques

## 8.3.1    Placing an oesophagostomy tube

This is an excellent technique for the provision of long-term critical nutrition, especially when the individual is difficult to handle for conventional stomach tubing; for example, giant species or very small juveniles.

As long as husbandry is adequate, placing an oesophagostomy (O) tube also enables more nursing at home than in the clinic.

Individuals can tolerate the tube for many weeks to months, although care must be taken to clean the insertion site as regularly as possible (though this may not be possible, given the original reasons for placing the tube).

Special care must be taken with aquatic species, as wound contamination is more likely, meaning that dry docking is essential when using this technique (see Chapter 3.3.4).

### Tube choice

Soft plastic or silicone tubes should be selected. The diameter should not exceed 50% of the oesophagus.

The tube should be pre-measured (and marked accordingly) to ensure that it reaches the stomach (approximately halfway between the head and the tail on the plastron) and leaving a sufficient tube length such that it can be secured to the carapace even when the head is retracted.

It is also important to measure the volume of water required to fill the tube – this will be needed to ensure adequate flushing of the tube after each feed, reducing the risk of tube blockage.

### Site

The neck just ventral to the ear scale and a quarter of the way between the ear scale and the thoracic inlet (nearer ear) – the oesophagus passes down the right side of the neck, so it is anatomically more correct to place the tube on that side. However, many will place the tube on the left side of the neck with no adverse consequences to the patient.

## Anaesthesia

Sedation (see Chapter 6) should be used except in debilitated individuals, where local anaesthetic infiltration of the incision site is used alone.

## Skin preparation

Skin should be prepared in the usual manner for sterile surgery – see Chapter 8.1.

## Technique

- Curved haemostats are inserted into the mouth, and the skin at the incision site is tented and incised over the tips of the haemostats. The haemostats are pushed through the skin (see Figure 8.3.1).
- A local anaesthetic splash block is applied to the incision.
- The tip of the O tube is grasped and withdrawn via the mouth (see Figure 8.3.2).
- The tube is doubled back and pushed down the oesophagus. The tube is inserted down the oesophagus until the pre-measured mark on the tube is reached.
- Inexperienced operators may prefer to radiograph the animal to confirm the tube position – for this reason, radio-opaque tubes should be used.
- The tube is secured to the skin using a Chinese finger trap suture, with non-absorbable or slowly absorbed suture material (see Figure 8.3.3).
- The exterior portion of the tube is secured to the carapace using an adhesive bandage. Sufficient length should be left such that the animal can withdraw its

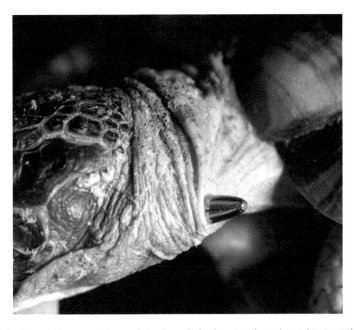

Figure 8.3.1    Curved haemostats are introduced via the mouth and used to tent the skin of the neck. An incision is made over the haemostat points and these are pushed through the skin. *Source*: Chitty, J. (2009) Oesophagostomy tubes in tortoises. *Companion Animal* 14(2), 80–82. © Mark Allen Holdings Limited.

head fully into the shell. However, the tube should be positioned so that it does not interfere with vision, or with movement of the foreleg.

- On recovery, if the animal is attempting to remove the tube by rubbing with the foreleg, a cohesive bandage may be placed over the large scales of the foreleg. If this is done, the bandage should be changed every 2–3 days and the limb checked for swelling. If the tube is difficult to maintain, it may be repositioned ventral to the forelimb and taped to the plastron, and thence to the carapace where it is finally secured.

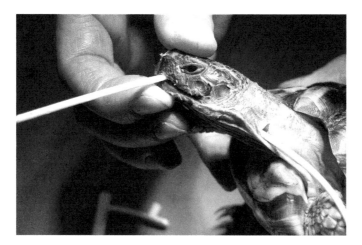

Figure 8.3.2   The oesophagostomy tube is grasped with the haemostats and pulled through into the mouth to the measured mark. It is then doubled back on itself and the tip of the tube pushed down the oesophagus into the stomach. *Source*: Chitty, J. (2009) Oesophagostomy tubes in tortoises. *Companion Animal* 14(2), 80–82. © Mark Allen Holdings Limited.

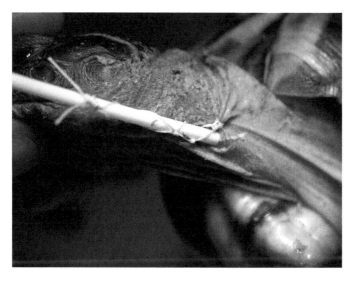

Figure 8.3.3   The tube is secured using a Chinese finger trap suture. *Source*: Chitty, J. (2009) Oesophagostomy tubes in tortoises. *Companion Animal* 14(2), 80–82. © Mark Allen Holdings Limited.

## Removal of the tube

This should be done when the animal has begun eating for itself (most animals are happy to eat with the tube in place).

Sedation is not always required, unless the tube insertion site cannot be accessed.

The suture is cut and the tube withdrawn. Any scab or reactive material should be removed.

The skin can then be glued.

## 8.3.2  Plastronotomy/Coeliotomy

- Plastronotomy provides access to the coelomic cavity, giving adequate exposure for most surgical procedures.
- Mark the incision area, taking care to stay cranial to the pelvis. This underlies the middle to caudal femoral scutes.
- Also avoid any hinges present in the species.
- Scrub the surgical site, especially along the suture lines where, especially in older animals, the surface is rough and it is difficult to prep.
- A high-speed saw is used to make the incision. One assistant holds the anaesthetised animal. Another drips saline on to the blade to dissipate heat and minimise thermal tissue damage.
- Angle the incision to create a bevelled edge that will fit tightly back in place without dropping through into the coelomic cavity. This gives good bone to bone apposition, promoting better healing.
- The caudal incision does not need to be completely transected, allowing the flap to be reflected caudally. This maintains a blood supply to the flap, giving better healing. Some surgeons completely transect the bone and remove the piece of bone, giving improved access.
- The hatch is reflected using a periosteal elevator, exposing the abdominal musculature, which is reflected to give access to the coelomic membrane with the bilateral paramedian ventral abdominal veins (see Figure 8.3.4).
- A midline incision is made, taking care to avoid the large ventral abdominal veins.
- Surgery of structures deep in the coelomic cavity can be difficult. Long-handled instruments, vascular clips and techniques borrowed from microsurgery and endoscopic surgery are often required (see Figure 8.3.5).
- On completion, it is important to suture the coelomic membrane. If the ventral abdominal veins are damaged, they can be ligated.
- The bone flap is slotted back in place. Make sure the edges are clean so that there is good bone to bone apposition. If the cut was straight, it should be a tight fit. Any gaps can be bridged with bone wax to prevent the sealant dripping between the segments of bone.
- Strips of mesh can be placed over the incisions and a rapidly drying epoxy resin applied to create a waterproof covering. Some surgeons apply the epoxy resin directly, without the mesh
- Keep the resin well clear of any hinges present in that species.

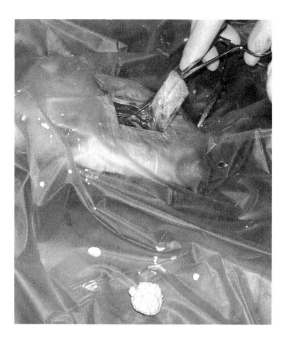

Figure 8.3.4    A large urolith removed by plastronotomy from a *G. sulcata*.

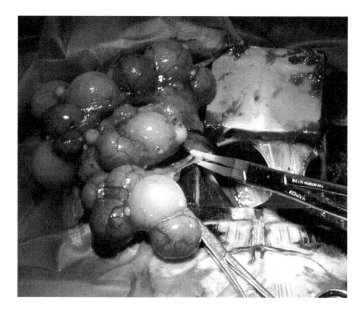

Figure 8.3.5    An ovariosalpingectomy via a plastronotomy.

- The patch will fall off in a few years, depending on the growth rate of the individual.
- Polymethyl methacrylate (PMMA) is the most commonly used resin. It is exothermic on curing, but if not applied in too thick a layer, this will not damage the underlying tissue.

- Analgesia is important. See Chapter 6.1 for systemic analgesics, and apply a topical splash block to the plastron incision wounds as detailed in Chapter 6.1.

## Juvenile individuals and pancake tortoises (*Malacochersus tornieri*)

- Juvenile individuals and Pancake tortoises with soft shells can have the incision made, with a blade, in the shape of a capital H on their side and the flaps reflected sidewards.
- The plastron is sutured closed. Gaps are bridged with bone wax. The whole area is covered with a layer of epoxy resin to form a waterproof seal that will fall off in time as the animal grows.

All staff in the operating area must wear protective goggles while the saw is incising the plastron. There is a risk of the blade shattering.

The combination of a high-speed saw, blood and the saline used as a coolant will result in nearby equipment, walls and ceilings being sprayed. Equipment should be covered with plastic sheets. Staff should wear protective aprons.

The saw must be of a type designed to dissipate heat rapidly. A new blade for each surgery is recommended, to achieve a clean cut.

### 8.3.3   Pre-femoral approach to coeliotomy

Pre-femoral coeliotomy gives access to:

- the urinary bladder
- the reproductive tract
- parts of the gastrointestinal system

It is also the approach for coelioscopy through a very small stab-incision.

- Access and visualisation of the coelomic cavity is much reduced and on some occasions a repeat surgery on the opposite side or a plastron osteotomy may be required.
- It is a less traumatic surgical approach.
- It may be less painful than plastron osteotomy.
- This approach provides access to the coelomic cavity without the need for plastron osteotomy and the creation of a bone flap.
- Coelioscopic assistance is commonly required with this approach, so it should only be used with the appropriate scopes on standby.
- General anaesthesia, appropriate analgesia and supportive care are required for surgery via the pre-femoral approach.
- In-depth anatomical knowledge is required for this approach, due to the reduced visibility.

- Positioning depends on the aims of the procedure.
- The hind limb is secured in extension to allow access to the pre-femoral fossa.
- In some species, the horn marginal scutes of the carapace can be burred a few millimetres back to provide greater access. Care needs to be taken not to expose bone. In less pigmented individuals, especially juveniles, the area can be trans-illuminated for better visualisation of where sensitive tissues start.
- Aseptic techniques must be strictly applied.

## *Technique*

- A craniocaudal skin incision is made in the centre of the pre-femoral fossa.
- The muscles are separated by blunt dissection.
- The coelomic membrane is incised to gain access to the coelomic cavity.
- The coelomic membrane, together with the muscle layer, is closed with either simple interrupted sutures or a continuous suture.
- The skin is closed with everting mattress sutures or skin staples.
- Surgical glue can be used to close the small incisions used for coelioscopy.

# 9   Clinical Pathology

## 9.1   Haematology and Serum Biochemistry

As described in Chapter 5.1, haematology and biochemistry are essential tools in the investigation of sick Chelonia.

Good-quality samples are essential and correct sample-taking is discussed in Chapter 5.1.

The following is a guide to the main parameters tested and their interpretation.

### Packed cell volume (PCV)

PCV is often reported as haematocrit (HCT), yet these are not the same. PCV is the physical measurement of the percentage of blood volume that is red blood cells. HCT is a calculated value for the same parameter. As these calculations use the smaller human red cell as the basis for the volume calculation, it is normal for the HCT to be slightly lower than PCV in chelonia. This is of little clinical significance other than when monitoring PCV or HCT in serial samples when it is vital to follow the same parameter to allow consistency.

- Raised:
  - hibernation
  - may be higher in males and in adults
  - dehydration

While PCV and total protein may rise in dehydrated individuals, many of these are also debilitated (usually causing a fall in PCV and proteins). In these cases, PCV and total protein may be lowered from normal, yet still artificially raised by

*Essentials of Tortoise Medicine and Surgery*, First Edition. John Chitty and Aidan Raftery.
© 2013 John Chitty and Aidan Raftery. Published 2013 by John Wiley & Sons, Ltd.

dehydration. This means that these are not always reliable indicators of dehydration (see below), and when other markers of dehydration are raised, the PCV and protein levels should be regarded as reading higher than they really are.

- Lowered:
  - may be lower in the middle of winter and summer
  - lower in females and juveniles
  - lowered by lymphodilution
  - poor nutrition/husbandry
  - blood loss
  - haemolysis
  - anaemia of chronic disease

## White cell count

- Raised:
  - hibernation
  - inflammatory response
- Lowered:
  - post-hibernation
  - lymphodilution
  - may also fall in infectious/inflammatory conditions where the animal is in poor condition or demand exceeds the production rate

## Heterophils

- Raised:
  - in summer
  - infectious/inflammatory response
  - stress
- Lowered:
  - in hibernation
  - may also fall in infectious/inflammatory conditions where the animal is in poor condition or demand exceeds the production rate

## Eosinophils

- Raised:
  - winter
  - parasitism
  - inflammatory disease – these cells modulate mast cell activity, and so will be seen where there is inflammation of mast cell-rich tissues (e.g. skin, gut, lung and uterus)

## Lymphocytes

- Raised:
  - summer
  - higher in females and juveniles
  - inflammation
  - lymphoproliferative disease
- Lowered:
  - fall in winter
  - lymphodilution
  - stress
  - chronic disease
  - malnutrition/anorexia

## Monocytes

May be raised in chronic infection/inflammatory conditions.

Many authors now regard azurophils and monocytes as being the same in chelonia – they are usually referred to as monocytes.

## Thrombocytes

May be used as pleuripotent stem cells and recruited into other cell lines.

May be lowered in malnutrition/chronic disease along with depression of other cell lines.

In some inflammatory conditions, these may be recruited into the general cell response and a phagocytic response may be seen in the thrombocytes.

## Total protein

- Raised:
  - breeding females
  - dehydration

While PCV and total protein may rise in dehydrated individuals, many of these are also debilitated (usually causing a fall in PCV and proteins). In these cases, PCV and total protein may be lowered from normal, yet still artificially raised by dehydration (see the PCV section).

Electrophoresis is recommended where protein/globulin levels are elevated. However, it should be borne in mind that interpretation is in its infancy and recent work suggests that some different changes may be seen in different groups of reptiles (Gimenez *et al.* 2010).

- Lowered:
  - lymphodilution
  - anorexia/malnutrition
  - liver disease
  - parasitism
  - chronic disease
  - enteropathy
  - nephropathy

## Albumin

- Raised:
  - higher in females – especially reproductively active
  - dehydration (see above)
- Lowered:
  - lymphodilution
  - anorexia/malnutrition
  - liver disease
  - parasitism
  - chronic disease
  - enteropathy
  - nephropathy
  - may be lower in immature animals

## Globulin

- Raised:
  - inflammatory response (albumin:globulin should be more than or equal to one)
  - breeding females
  - if raised, electrophoresis may be useful (see above)
  - may be raised with albumin in dehydration
- Lowered:
  - lymphodilution

## Alkaline phosphatase (ALKP)

Found generally in tissues – not specific to any particular organ.
May be raised with any tissue damage.
Specifically, may be part of the pattern seen in female reproductive activity.

## Alanine transaminase (ALT)

Found generally in tissues – not specific to any organ.

May be raised in renal disease due to reduced renal excretion.

Rise may be part of the pattern seen in female reproductive activity.

## Aspartate transaminase (AST)

Found generally in tissues – not specific to any particular organ.

May be raised with any tissue damage.

It has been suggested that this may be raised with CK in cardiac disease.

## Creatinine kinase (CK)

Found generally in tissues – not specific to any particular organ.

May be raised with any tissue damage – rapid rise and short half-life in plasma following tissue/muscle trauma, including after venipuncture/intramuscular injection of irritant drugs.

It has been suggested that this may be raised with AST in cardiac disease.

## Gamma glutamyl transferase (GGT)

In other species, release from the biliary tree in bile stasis.

Less specific in chelonians and more a marker of tissue damage.

May be raised in renal disease, as associated with the nephron however, it tends to be released into the urine rather than the circulation.

## Glutamate dehydrogenase (GLDH)

Raised in hepatocellular damage – considered specific for this, though not very sensitive.

## Lactate dehydrogenase (LDH)

Found generally in tissues – not specific to any particular organ.

May be raised with any tissue damage.

Raised in haemolysis.

## Beta-hydroxybutyrate (BHB)

This is a marker of ketogenesis and so is an important assessment in anorexic/depleted individuals.

Ketosis indicates an important need to provide critical nutrition.

## Bile acids

Significantly elevated levels (from 48-hour fasted individuals) appear to be associated with liver function disorders.

Mildly elevated levels are hard to interpret, as are those from non-fasted animals.

## Total calcium

A measure of protein-bound inactive calcium and physiologically active ionised calcium.

Total calcium may be raised in reproductively active females.

Lowered total calcium may be seen artificially (i.e. not truly hypocalcaemic) when protein levels are lowered. Therefore ionised calcium should also be assessed especially, as it is less affected by reproductive status and not affected by lymphodilution.

Calcium levels may be lowered in nutritional deficiency, renal disease, Vitamin D3 deficiency and lack of ultraviolet light.

It should always be assessed with phosphate and protein levels.

## Phosphate

Raised in haemolysis.

May be raised in renal disease (though the calcium:phosphate ratio, generally 1.5–2, is less reliable a measure of renal function than in other reptiles).

Raised in reproductively active females (though the calcium:phosphate ratio is maintained).

Higher in juveniles.

Raised in nutritional secondary hyperparathyroidism.

Lowered in anorexia/malnutrition – not affected by lymphodilution.

## Cholesterol

Raised in females in summer.
Raised in hepatic lipidosis.
Lowered in malnutrition.

## Triglycerides

Raised in reproductively active females.
Lowered pre-hibernation.

## Glucose

Rises post-hibernation.
May see transient stress hyperglycaemia associated with sampling.

Some suggest that it may be raised in pancreatic disease.

Lowered in:

- anorexia/malnutrition
- depleted animals
- liver disease
- chronic disease

## Electrolytes

Electrolytes should always be measured either immediately on whole blood/
  plasma, or if delayed then plasma should be separated immediately – heparin
  gel tubes are best.
Otherwise, even small amounts of post-sampling haemolysis will affect the
  results.
Electrolytes tend to be unaffected by lymphodilution.

## Sodium

Raised:

- higher post-hibernation
- reduced water intake/increased losses

Lowered:

- haemolysis/post-sampling in whole blood

## Potassium

Raised:

- haemolysis
- higher in April to August
- renal disease – an important prognostic indicator (see later)
- dehydration

Lowered:

- enteropathy and renal disease

## Urea

Raised:

- Dehydration – an excellent measure in terrestrial species, as it indicates the degree to which the animal is drawing on bladder water stores.
- Renal disease – other than as a measure of dehydration, this is not a sensitive indicator of renal disease.
- Post-prandial effects in carnivorous species – may be seen for 24–48 hours post-feeding, so should be assessed after a period of starvation.

Unaffected by lymphodilution.

## Uric acid

Raised:

- Lipaemia.
- Excess dietary protein (or post-prandial effects in carnivorous species – may be seen for 24–48 hours post-feeding, so should be assessed after a period of starvation).
- Dehydration.
- Renal disease.

Lowered:

- Lymphodilution.
- Liver disease.
- Malnutrition in carnivorous species.

## Various effects

- Hibernation:
  - ○ rise in hibernation – PCV, white cell count, eosinophils
  - ○ fall in hibernation – heterophils, lymphocytes, potassium
- Spring:
  - ○ rise post-hibernation – heterophils, lymphocytes, cholesterol, glucose, potassium
  - ○ fall post-hibernation – PCV, white cell count, eosinophils, sodium
- Age:
  - ○ adults have –
    - ■ higher – PCV, albumin
    - ■ lower – lymphocytes, phosphate, triglycerides, cholesterol
- Sex:
  - ○ Males have –
    - ■ higher – PCV
    - ■ lower – lymphocytes, albumin, cholesterol

- Reproductive activity in females:
  - ○ ALT, ALKP, CK, total protein, globulin, albumin, total calcium, phosphate, triglycerides and cholesterol may all rise in the reproductively active female
- Haemolysis:
  - ○ potassium, phosphate and tissue enzymes may all *rise* in haemolysed samples
  - ○ sodium and ionised calcium may *fall* in haemolysed samples
- Lymphodilution – the following fall in lymphodiluted samples:
  - ○ PCV, red cell counts, all white cell parameters/counts and protein parameters

**NB** The clinical pathologist may be able to detect lymphodilution on blood smears, as there may be a blue proteinaceous background.

## Cell cytology

As in other exotic species, white cell counts may not always rise in inflammatory conditions – indeed, these may actually fall especially in run-down or depleted (see Chapter 10 for definition) individuals (see Figures 9.1.1, 9.1.2, 9.1.3 and 9.1.4).

However, changes in cell morphology will give a far better indication of inflammatory status:

- Toxicity – toxic changes may be seen in heterophils and/or monocytes. Indicates active inflammatory response, usually to bacterial infections.

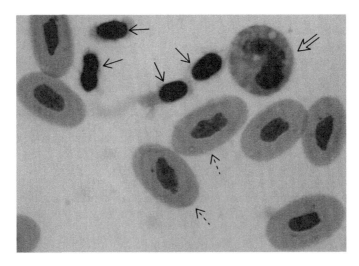

Figure 9.1.1    Thrombocytes (→) – note that they are nucleated. These may be hard to distinguish from lymphocytes, but in general are slightly more ovoid and have more obvious cytoplasm. These may be observed phagocytosing bacteria in an inflammatory response. The cell on the right is a monocyte (⟹) – the numbers of these cells may be raised (or there may be a relative monocytosis) in chronic and/or granulomatous inflammatory reactions. Red blood cells (--») shown for relative size. Courtesy of Nick Carmichael, CTDS Lab Ltd.

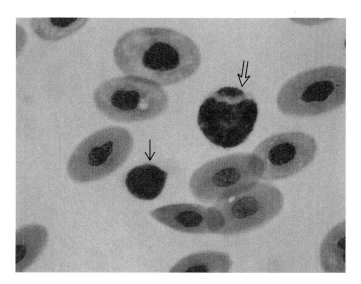

Figure 9.1.2   Heterophil (upper right ⇒) of the white cells and active monocyte (→). Courtesy of Nick Carmichael, CTDS Lab Ltd.

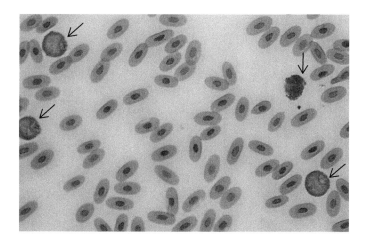

Figure 9.1.3   Eosinophils (→) seen amongst red cells. One cell is slightly disrupted in preparation. Eosinophils are believed to modulate mast cell/basophil reactions. They are therefore often raised in inflammatory conditions affecting mast cell-rich tissues; for example, gut, skin and lungs. This includes, but is not exclusive to, parasitic infections. Courtesy of Nick Carmichael, CTDS Lab Ltd.

- Phagocytosis – may be seen in heterophils, monocytes, lymphocytes and/or thrombocytes (see Figure 9.1.5). Again, this indicates a response to bacterial infection – usually systemic or septicaemic infection.
- Left shift – rarely seen in heterophils or monocytes. However, release of juvenile cells shows an inflammatory response.

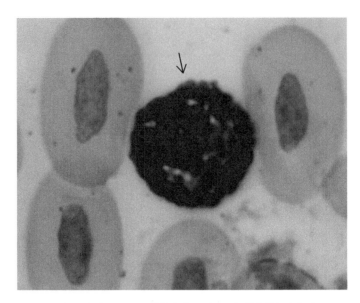

Figure 9.1.4    Basophil (→). Courtesy of Nick Carmichael, CTDS Lab Ltd.

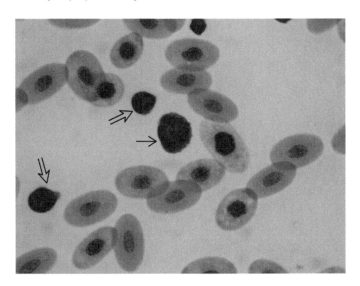

Figure 9.1.5    Reactive lymphocyte (→). Heterophil (⇒). Courtesy of Nick Carmichael, CTDS Lab Ltd.

Unusual cells may be seen in lymphoproliferative disease. However, this is extremely rare and the finding of unusual or dividing circulating white cells is more usually a sign of an extreme inflammatory response.

In anaemia, interpretation is similar to other species, with anaemia being classified as follows:

- Regenerative – may be seen following blood loss and haemolysis or in recovery from disease or depletion or hibernation (see Figure 9.1.6).

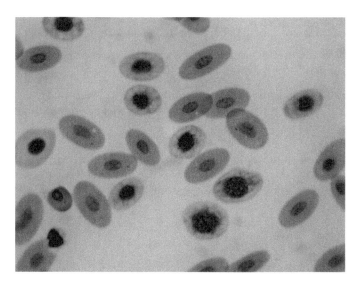

Figure 9.1.6    Polychromasia seen in red cells – indicative of a regenerative response in anaemia. Courtesy of Nick Carmichael, CTDS Lab Ltd.

Table 9.1.1    Prognostic Indicators in debilitated *Testudo* species

| Parameter | Action | Poor prognosis | Hopeless prognosis |
|---|---|---|---|
| Urea | > 2.1 mmol/l | > 10 | > 100 |
| Uric acid | > 400 µmol/l | > 1000 | > 2500 |
| Potassium (spun sample or patientside) | > 5 mmol/l | > 9 | |
| Ca:P – both raised in correct ratio | Depends – probably indicates reproductive activity in female: check albumin and total protein results | | |
| Ca:P | < 2:1 – may show renal disease | P > Ca | If P > Ca and fails to respond to oral phosphate binder plus fluids |

- Non-regenerative – may be seen as failure of cell production: bone marrow disease, malabsorption, malnutrition, parasitism or in severely depleted individuals (especially post-hibernation).

Other red cell parameters – mean cell volume, mean cellular haemoglobin concentration and so on – can be interpreted as in other species and provide further information regarding type, severity and recovery in anaemic individuals (see Latimer *et al.* 2003).

## Prognostic indicators

Table 9.1.1 may be useful in anorexic or depleted *Testudo* species, where dehydration and renal disease appear common.

In carnivorous species, urea and uric acid levels this high may be normal postprandial. In anorexic individuals (>48 hours), these levels may still be relevant.

Raised urea in the presence of normal uric acid indicates dehydration.

Raised uric acid with normal urea may show renal disease or dehydration (especially where the bladder has been emptied – urea levels appear to be an indication of water resorption from bladder water stores)

## References

Gimenenz, M., Saco, Y., Pato, R., Busquets, A., Martorell, J.M. & Bassols, A. (2010) Plasma protein electrophoresis of *Trachemys scripta* and *Iguana iguana*. *Veterinary Clinical Pathology*, 39(2), 227–235.

Latimer, K.S., Mahaffey, E.A. & Prasse, K.W. (eds) (2003) *Duncan & Prasse's Veterinary Laboratory Medicine: Clinical Pathology*, 4th edn, Iowa State University Press, Ames, IA.

# 9.2  Parasitology

The identification, life cycles and control of the common parasites of chelonia are described in Chapters 28 and 29.

This section covers the basic investigation of parasitic disease and means of collecting samples for parasitological investigation.

## Ectoparasites

See Chapter 28.

Generally, ectoparasites are readily identified with the naked eye. However, all cases of skin irritation should be thoroughly examined using magnification.

If in doubt, parasites may be collected on acetate strips and examined under a microscope, or preserved in alcohol and submitted to an entomological laboratory for examination.

In the United Kingdom (UK), parasites may be submitted to the parasitology department of the University of Liverpool Veterinary School (http://pcwww.liv.ac.uk/testapet/) for identification.

## Endoparasites

Endoparasitism is seen much more commonly than ectoparasitism as a cause of clinical disease in the UK – see Chapter 29.

Faecal examination for endoparasites should be undertaken in all cases of:

- lethargy
- weight loss/failure to gain weight
- anorexia
- diarrhoea/regurgitation
- secondary infection
- ileus or excess gas in the intestine
- prolapsed bowel

## Obtaining a faecal sample

This is not always straightforward, especially in the anorexic animal.

If the tortoise is passing faeces, then the owner should be instructed to bring in as fresh a sample as possible. Where this may be delayed more than 48 hours, the sample should be stored in a fridge in a sealed pot. Sometimes it may be worth adding a tiny amount of isotonic saline to keep the sample moist and wrapping the sample in cling film if there is likely to be a long delay, or the sample is to be posted in very hot weather.

Otherwise, samples may be obtained by:

- Bathing – warm water baths encourage defecation. Because of the dilution factor caused by the bath, these samples, if loose, will be unsuitable for quantitative analysis. If very loose, the animal should be watched and the sample syringed from the bath water immediately it is passed.
- Cloacal wash – warmed saline (at a rate of 10–15 ml/kg) may be gently syringed into the cloaca. This may encourage defecation or a small sample may be removed by syringe. These are rarely sufficient for more than a wet preparation for protozoa, rather than nematode ovum analysis – certainly a cloacal wash sample that is negative for nematode ova cannot be regarded as a true negative: in these cases, retesting is indicated as soon as a larger sample can be obtained.

**NB** Urine obtained by either of these methods may also be useful for assessing coccidians.

Faecal samples should be examined by the following methods.

## Direct wet preparation

A drop of faeces may be placed on a slide with a drop of warmed isotonic saline and covered with a cover slip. These preparations are good for monitoring numbers and type of motile protozoa. They should be examined as soon as possible after passage – ideally within 30 minutes. It is important to understand the relevance of motile protozoa (see Chapter 29). Many are normal in small numbers and the finding of no, or very few, trichomonads (and, especially, *Nyctotherus*) is highly significant, as a lack may result in maldigestion. Similarly, an overgrowth with vast numbers of motile protozoa may indicate an altered gastrointestinal environment and maldigestion. Wet preparations may also be useful for monitoring coccidians and nematodes if present in high numbers. High numbers of motile bacteria may also be noted and may be of significance in some cases.

## Faecal flotation

Standard zinc sulphate flotation techniques will be appropriate in Chelonia. Quantitative, semi-quantitative and qualitative methods are available, and the choice depends on the sensitivity required.

## Direct stains

Trichrome stains (e.g. 'Diff Quik', Dade) may be appropriate for identification of bacteria and yeast. For certain protozoa – for example, Cryptosporidia – modified Ziehl–Nielson stains may be used.

## Submission to external laboratories

Samples may be submitted to external laboratories and should be submitted in the same manner as for other species.

It is important to liaise with the laboratory prior to submission, to ensure that they are experienced and familiar with reptile parasitology, with respect to recognition of parasites and understanding of their clinical significance.

## Haemoparasites

Examinations for these rely on stained blood smears, and should be submitted to an experienced reptile haematologist/parasitologist. Each laboratory will have individual preferences and these should be discussed with the laboratory prior to submission. If in doubt, unstained fresh (no anti-coagulant) blood smears should be submitted – ideally, several slides with some thin smears and some thick.

## Further reading

For individual parasites, see Chapters 28 and 29.
The following may be of assistance in parasite recognition:

Barnard, S.M. & Upton, S.J. (1994) *A Veterinary Guide to the Parasites of Reptiles*, vol. 1, *Protozoa*. Krieger, Malabar, FL.

Barnard, S.M. & Upton, S.J. (2000) *A Veterinary Guide to the Parasites of Reptiles*, vol. 2, *Arthropods (Excluding Mites)*. Krieger, Malabar, FL.

Campbell, T.W. & Ellis, C.K. (2007) *Avian & Exotic Animal Hematology and Cytology*, 3rd edn. Blackwell Publishing, Oxford.

Greiner, E.C. & Mader, D.R. (2006) Parasitology. In: *Reptile Medicine and Surgery* (ed. D.R. Mader), 2nd edn, pp. 343–364. Saunders; St Louis, MO.

Hawkey, C.M. & Dennett, T.B. (1989) *A Colour Atlas of Comparative Veterinary Haematology*. Wolfe Medical Publications, Ipswich.

Jacobsen, E.R. (2007) Parasites and parasitic diseases of reptiles. In: *Infectious Diseases and Pathology of Reptiles* (ed. E.R. Jacobsen), pp. 571–666. Taylor & Francis, Boca Raton, FL.

McArthur, S., Wilkinson, R. & Meyer, J. (2004) *Medicine and Surgery of Tortoises and Turtles*. Blackwell, Oxford.

# 9.3 Microbiology

In general, bacterial disease is more common than fungal and sampling should be biased towards this.

However, fungal disease does occur (and is relatively more common in some parts of the world than the UK) and so should not be disregarded.

It is important to note that few agents can be considered primary pathogens other than in immunocompromised or naive animals. The role of underlying disease and poor husbandry in the aetiology of bacterial/fungal disease cannot be overstated in chelonia and must always be addressed.

Certain bacterial species may be considered more pathogenic than others. More pathogenic species are those that are most capable of causing infection in otherwise healthy animals and, hence, are those most likely to be isolated from lesions. In general, Gram-negative rods appear more likely to be involved in lesions/disease than Gram-positive cocci. However, this may reflect the role of opportunists from gut or environment. Certainly Gram-positive bacteria and anaerobes must be addressed when treating conditions where they may have gained entry – for example, post-dog bite.

However, most bacteria associated with disease are still likely to originate from normal commensal populations (especially in the gut) or from the environment. Therefore 'screening' procedures and prophylactic antibiosis cannot be recommended as a means of eradicating potentially 'pathogenic' species. Similarly, diagnosis of a bacterial-related disease should prompt further investigation of underlying disease and/or husbandry problems, especially where bacteria of relatively low pathogenicity are isolated.

Infections may range from acute to (more commonly) chronic granulomatous lesions, often with abscess production.

However, infection may disseminate to other organ systems especially by haematogenous spread. This means that even small localised lesions have the potential to cause systemic illness if left untreated.

## Septicaemia/bacteraemia

**Septicaemia** Systemic disease associated with the presence and persistence of bacteria (or their toxins) in the blood.

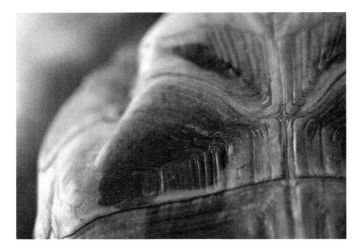

Figure 9.3.1   A typical shell petechiation in a tortoise with septicaemia. Pressing these areas of the shell with a fingernail will result in temporary localised blanching.

**Bacteraemia** The temporary presence of bacteria in the blood. These are not associated with clinical signs, but may cause embolic infections. In fact, this may be normal in healthy chelonia.

Septicaemia may occur as an acute condition following inoculation of bacteria into the animal via the skin or through the gut, or as a more chronic situation where localised infection has gone unnoticed or has not been adequately treated.

Clinical signs may be non-specific (lethargy, anorexia, weakness progressing to collapse and death), but may include signs of embolic infection; for example, polyarthritis, endocarditis and skin petechiae (shell and skin) or multiple shell/skin ulcerations (see Figure 9.3.1).

Where any bacterial disease is suspected, especially where petechiae are present or where there are multiple sites of infection or abscesses, the heart should be auscultated using an 8 MHz Doppler probe. The finding of a harsh murmur typical of endocarditis indicates a poor or grave prognosis.

Diagnosis of septicaemia is difficult. Blood culture is of little use, as bacteraemia may be common in reptiles and there is difficulty in obtaining samples without skin contamination. Haematology may show raised, normal or low total white cell counts. However, heterophils and/or macrophages will normally show toxicity and phagocytosed bacteria may be visible. This latter change should be differentiated from the finding of 'free' bacteria within the blood smear with no evidence of phagocytosis or toxic changes in the white cells; this may represent bacterial contamination of the sample or bacteraemia.

## Clinical approach

In general, where bacterial disease is suspected, lesions should be sampled and specimens tested in the following manner.

## *Cytology*

Aspirates can be smeared on slides or direct impression smears of open lesions can be examined. A trichrome stain (e.g. 'Diff Quik', Dade) should be used, although a Gram stain can be useful in differentiating some bacterial species. The finding of inflammatory cells is always suggestive of infection and bacteria may be directly visualised. Obviously, a sparse mixed population of bacteria suggests contamination or commensal organisms, whereas many monomorphic forms suggest greater significance, especially where Gram-negative rods are seen. This enables a rapid provisional diagnosis and prompt 'first guess' antibiosis based on bacterial morphology.

## *Culture and sensitivity*

A swab should be submitted from any bacterial lesions for bacteriological culture and sensitivity testing. Culture should be performed at 37°C and 22°C. This is because many of these organisms (of environmental origin) have adapted to grow at lower temperatures than those normally used. Similarly, culture in both aerobic and anaerobic/micro-aerophilic conditions should be used, as many of these organisms are adapted to lower oxygen concentrations. Rather than these culture requirements reflecting conditions found in the normal reptile, they reflect why the 'cold' or 'hypoxic' reptile is more vulnerable to bacterial infection. Sensitivity tests are essential, as antibiotic resistance is commonly encountered. Contamination by environmental or faecal bacteria makes interpretation very difficult. Swabs should always be taken from deeper parts of the lesion in order to avoid confusion with environmental contaminants. Blood culture techniques can be used, but the results must be interpreted with care because of the potential for a 'normal' bacteraemia. In all cases, haematology should also be used to assist in differentiating between bacteraemia and septicaemia (see above). The other problem with blood culture is that it is much more difficult to take a sample without contamination by skin bacteria, compared to the situation in mammals. Also, biopsy samples may be submitted for culture – this is especially useful for shell lesions where deeper samples may be submitted after debridement for bacterial and fungal culture.

## *Histopathology*

This will reveal organisms and the cellular response to them, which may help to distinguish infection from contamination.

Although systemic antibiosis is generally important to avoid embolic spread or septicaemia, surgery is often required to remove bacterial lesions.

## Salmonella

These organisms have a variable degree of pathogenicity in reptiles. They are often normal inhabitants of the reptile gut; hence their frequent appearance as invading agents in lesions or in a gut dysbiosis/overgrowth.

A number of species have been implicated as pathogens causing septicaemia, pneumonia, coelomitis, abscess, granuloma, hypovolaemic shock and death, although the vast majority of these have also been isolated from healthy reptiles, reinforcing the feeling that these are opportunistic pathogens. The potential pathogenicity will vary according to the critical number of organisms required to cause disease, the current state of the host's immune system and the location of the bacterial entry relative to their normal 'position' in the body.

Although not a significant hazard to the reptile, these species may constitute a significant zoonotic risk. Accordingly, a lot of research has been undertaken to establish screening methods and/or methods of producing *Salmonella*-free reptiles. To date, these have appeared to be unsuccessful, and generalised use of disinfectants and antibiotics in the reptile or in the environment of aquatic species cannot be recommended. Care should also be taken with the use of antibiotics for other bacterial infections, as these drugs will also affect the normal gut bacteria, including *Salmonella* spp., and may result in the development of antibiotic resistance.

The standard means of diagnosis is culture, although it is fairly insensitive and so should not be used as a screening test. All reptiles should be considered carriers.

## Human reptile-associated salmonellosis

For the reasons outlined above, this is a potential problem where humans and chelonians are in contact. Nonetheless, it is only a significant risk to immuno-compromised people and does not overall preclude the keeping of these species as pets.

Screening and prophylactic therapy are not appropriate for controlling *Salmonella* levels in Chelonia, so the emphasis must be on handlers to reduce contamination.

Excellent guides to this are produced by Defra (UK) and the Association of Reptile and Amphibian Veterinarians.

In essence:

- Always wash hands with hot soapy water after handling chelonians or equipment associated with them, or when handling/defrosting food for carnivorous species.
- Do not kiss chelonians or share food.
- Do not have chelonians in food preparation areas or in bathrooms, especially where children bathe. Kitchen and bathroom sinks should not be used for bathing chelonians or for cleaning associated equipment.
- Do not eat, drink or smoke while handling chelonians or cleaning out enclosures.
- Waste material or water used for cleaning enclosures should not be disposed of via a sink – the toilet is more appropriate.

- Children under five or immunocompromised individuals should not handle chelonians. Older children should only handle chelonians when supervised by an adult, to ensure strict hygiene.
- Keep chelonians as healthy as possible to reduce shedding of salmonellae.

In the hospital situation, stressed ill chelonians are very likely to be shedding salmonellae. This enhances the need to maintain strict barrier nursing for all sick chelonians.

In addition, examination gloves should be worn by staff handling chelonians, especially aquatic species.

## Mycobacteriosis

This is also a potential zoonosis, as Mycobacteria Other Than Tuberculous (MOTT) mycobacteria are found in lesions in reptiles. Typically, these lesions resemble human disease, with tubercles found in many different organs. Clinical signs relate to the location of the lesions, but often include lethargy and wasting. The species typically found include *Mycobacterium avium-complex* (MAC), *M. marinum*, *M. chelonae*, *M. fortuitum*, *M. smegmatis*, *M. phamnopheos* and *M. phlei*.

These infections are rare in chelonians, but should not be disregarded.

Suspicion should be aroused on finding typical granulomatous lesions, especially those that do not respond to antibiotic therapy (see Figures 22.3 and 22.4).

Samples (aspirates, biopsies or excised lesions) should be submitted for acid-fast staining. If positive, culture may be attempted.

There is no recommended therapy, and in view of the zoonotic potential of these organisms, euthanasia of the affected animal is generally an appropriate course of action unless there is a single localised lesion that may be completely excised.

In-contact animals should be screened and vivaria used by the affected animal disposed of rather than used for a different animal.

When a suspected case is being hospitalised in the hospital, it should be barrier nursed and great care used when handling it, to avoid human infection.

## Mycoplasmosis

Mycoplasmosis has emerged as a major factor in respiratory disease of Chelonia.

In tortoises, it is one of the components and causes of the Upper Respiratory Tract Disease (URTD) complex. It has also been reported as a cause of pneumonia.

The major species involved is *Mycoplasma agassizii* and it has been isolated from a range of species. While transmission studies in desert and gopher tortoises have shown that this agent does fulfil Koch's Postulates and may be considered a potential primary pathogen, it should be noted that this agent may also be detected in clinically normal tortoises. Pathogenicity may, therefore, also depend on the host species, the strain of the agent and the health/immune status of the host (see Chapters 23 and 24).

Diagnosis may be carried out using the following methods.

## Culture of the organism

Specific culture and transport media should be used and the laboratory should be contacted prior to sending the sample. Ideally, a specialised laboratory should be used; for example, Mycoplasma Experience, UK.

## Serology

An ELISA test has been developed for this species. Although specific monoclonal antibodies are used, there may be cross-reactions with other tortoise antibodies, and levels of antibody appear to fluctuate with season. As with all serological tests, a positive reaction merely indicates exposure, not the presence of the organism.

## Polymerase chain reaction (PCR)

PCR for mycoplasmal antigen is appropriate for swabs taken from the mouth. This should be more sensitive than culture and indicates the presence of the organism in lesions. It has also shown carriage of organisms in clinically normal tortoise mouths; and in one study the presence of mycoplasmal antigen could not be correlated with the presence of lesions, which may indicate that this organism is a part of the normal tortoise oral flora or, more likely, that latent infection is common and that even 'healthy' tortoises may be regarded as carriers. This study also suggested that Horsfield's tortoises may be more likely to be associated with this organism (Soares *et al.* 2003).

## Fungi

Systemic mycoses are much less common than bacterial infections. Nevertheless, they are considerably more common in reptiles than in endotherms.

It is therefore important for the clinician to take samples for mycological as well as bacteriological tests, especially when there has been an apparent 'antibiotic failure'.

As with bacteria, fungi rarely act as primary pathogens, with infection representing opportunistic infection of the compromised reptile from the environment. However, *Fusarium incarnatum* infections of the skin/carapace of gopher tortoises have appeared to be primary infections, with no underlying causes being readily apparent (Rose *et al.* 2001). Otherwise, it is extremely unusual to see 'outbreaks' of fungal disease, even where there are shared husbandry problems.

Species isolated most frequently include *Aspergillus* spp., *Mucor* spp., *Candida* spp., *Penicillum* spp., *Paecilomyces* spp., *Fusarium* spp., *Acremonium* spp. and *Geotrichum* spp. Mixed fungal infections may also be found.

'Typical' lesions include granulomata, although they may also commonly be associated with 'shell rot', and ulcerative skin/shell lesions in aquatic species.

Signs of systemic mycoses relate to whether disease is caused by invasion of tissue or release of toxins from more localised lesions or by ingestion of contaminated foodstuffs (mycotoxicosis). For this latter reason, even small localised lesions should be viewed seriously.

Systemic mycoses generally originate from the respiratory or gastrointestinal systems. Clinical signs relate to the organ system principally affected. Signs may only be seen when disease is already advanced.

## Diagnostics

Ideally, samples from lesions (aspirates, scrapes, swabs or biopsies) should be submitted to a specialist laboratory for fungal culture. However, it may difficult to isolate fungi due to their sensitive nature/culture needs or due to overgrowth of environmental bacteria/fungi contaminants. Samples should, therefore, be taken from deep within lesions. This is particularly important for cutaneous lesions, especially chelonian shells.

Culture may also take a long time, which may hamper diagnosis, especially as many of these diseases will be well advanced by the time of presentation.

More rapid diagnosis may be facilitated by submission of biopsy samples for histopathology or of aspirates, smears or fluid exudates/washes for cytological examination where fungal organisms may be seen.

It should be noted that special staining (e.g. Periodic Acid Schiff or silver stain) may be required to identify fungal hyphae, so the pathologist should always be advised when fungal disease is suspected. H&E stains will not always stain fungal hyphae.

## Virology

Viruses associated with disease in Chelonia include the following:

- herpesvirus
- iridovirus
- papillomavirus
- reovirus
- paramyxovirus
- picornavirus
- togavirus – West Nile virus
- circovirus (one case reported in *Chrysemys*)

As with bacteria and fungi, underlying factors such as husbandry and stressors (e.g. mixing individuals/species) may well be associated with immunocompromise, allowing viral disease to take over.

Nonetheless, exposure of naive individuals to novel viruses can result in 'primary' viral disease and outbreaks.

The gold standard for all viral disease is isolation. However, this may be expensive and time-consuming, and false negatives certainly occur.

The following may also be considered:

- Polymerase Chain Reaction (PCR) – appropriate for herpesvirus in tortoises. Plain swabs should be taken from the pharynx and oral cavity.
- Histopathology.
- Electron microscopy.

Serology may also be available for herpesvirus, paramyxovirus, togavirus and picornavirus. However, this indicates exposure, not necessarily disease. Therefore it may be of restricted use (other than rule-out) in clinical cases and of far more use in screening quarantined individuals before entry to virus-negative colonies.

The diagnostic tests available do vary considerably from country to country and so it is essential to speak to a diagnostic laboratory before submitting samples.

## References

Rose, F.L., Koke, J., Koehn, R., *et al.* (2001) Identification of the etiological agent for necrotizing scute disease in the Texas tortoise. *Journal of Wildlife Diseases*, 37, 223–228.

Soares, J.F., Chalker, V.J., Erles, K., Holtby, S., Waters, M. & McArthur, S. (2003) Prevalence of *Mycoplasma agassizii* and chelonian Herpesvirus in captive tortoises (*Testudo* spp.) in the United Kingdom. In: *Proceedings of the 10th Annual Conference of the Association of Reptilian & Amphibian Veterinarians*, Minneapolis, 4–9 October 1991.

# 9.4 Post-mortem Examination Techniques

Record keeping and documentation are very important aspects of the post-mortem examination. Familiarity with the normal anatomy of the species under examination is vitally important in order to be able to recognise abnormalities. The post mortem should be carried out meticulously and tissues examined in a predetermined sequence. Careful preparation before starting is essential to obtaining maximum benefit.

## Preparation

1. Collect the necessary equipment:

   - Gloves, rubber or latex, and a surgical mask plus appropriate clothing.
   - Hacksaw, screwdriver, bone cutters, scalpel, rat tooth forceps, scissors, tissue probe, Bunsen burner or lighter, swabs and paper towels.
   - Camera, ruler, callipers, Gram scales, plus a means of recording findings.
   - Culture swabs, labels, formalin pots, microscope slides and containers for various samples, such as freezing tissue samples, faecal samples, stomach contents and so on.

2. Review the medical and husbandry history:

   - The environment and diet need to be evaluated thoroughly.
   - Details of any contact with other animals, either of the same of different species, and the health of these animals can give valuable clues.
   - The medical history includes details of clinical signs and symptoms prior to death, the available clinicopathological information (haematology, biochemistry values etc.), imaging data (e.g. radiographs and ultrasonograms), and treatments administered and their observed effects.
   - In addition, any information on the possibility of trauma or any possible exposure to toxins could be vital.

3. Collect biological data:

   - Weight, straight carapace length, curved carapace length, straight width, curved width and height.

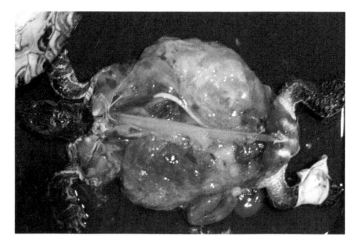

Figure 9.4.1   The shell is removed. The right lung is grossly abnormal.

- Scan for microchips.
- Photograph.

4.  External examination:

- Confirmation of species identity.
- Skin and shell evaluation.
- Body condition scoring.
- Degree of hydration.
- Evidence of trauma.
- Swellings.
- Any other abnormalities found externally.

5.  Preparing for internal examination:

- The bridges are cut using the hacksaw or similar.
- Cut the skin with either scissors or a scalpel blade at its attachments to the plastron.
- The plastron can then be lifted from the rear and its soft tissue attachments bluntly dissected until the plastron can be lifted free.
- Incise the coelomic membrane to collect a sample from the liver for culture and sensitivity.
- Remove the carapace by incising skin around the margin and disarticulating from its attachments to the cervical and coccygeal vertebrae on its internal surface, using a screwdriver or similar.
- The carcase, now minus the shell, is then placed in ventral recumbency (see Figure 9.4.1).

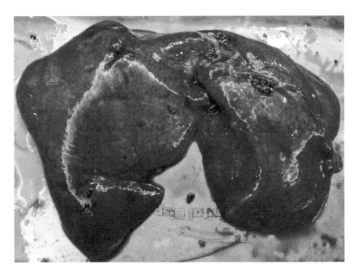

Figure 9.4.2    The liver, with parasitic tracts.

6. Internal examination:

- Incise the lung wall and collect a sample for culture.
- Locate the thyroid and remove it, including enough tissue to include the parathyroid, thymus and ultimobrachial bodies.
- Incise the pericardial sac. Evaluate the heart and remove to examine, including the chambers and valves.
- Remove the lungs and spread out before opening both sides. Collect samples of any abnormalities.
- Turn over the carcase and examine the liver. Remove from carcase and collect samples from any abnormalities (see Figure 9.4.2).
- Identify the spleen, remove and incise, collecting samples from any abnormality.
- Record if the bladder is full or empty, and the presence of any stones and so forth.
- Identify both adrenals and sample if abnormal.
- Incise the kidneys to check the pelvis. Sample if abnormal.
- Confirm the sex of the individual. Identify and sample if necessary ovaries (record ovarian activity) and oviducts in the female and the testis, epididymis and vas deferens (record if in breeding condition).
- Next, examine the gastrointestinal tract. Gut contents from different areas should be collected for separate examination and the gross appearance of the lining evaluated. Start with the oral cavity and work down the oesophagus, stomach, duodenum and pancreas, ileum and jejunum, caecum and colon, and finish with the rectum and cloaca.
- Remove the brain from the head and evaluate the spinal cord on the ventral surface of the carapace. If necessary, the whole head can be submitted for

histology, but some skin and bone needs to be removed to allow proper preservation of the tissues.
- The last tissue sampled is bone marrow, which can be collected from the pelvis and the gular projections.

7. Completion:

- Label and freeze the carcase.
- Process the samples.
- Check the written record of the examination for accuracy and completeness. Clean and disinfect instruments used and any surfaces contaminated during the examination, including areas such as door handles and water taps.

# ▋▋ Presentations

# 10 Anorexia

Anorexia is defined as a lack or loss of appetite.

In reptiles, it can be hard to differentiate the pathological state from the physical, as animals may normally not eat every day (and many authorities recommend not feeding every day) or may stop eating for periods when entering or emerging from hibernation, or when showing reproductive activity (digging/egg laying in females; hyperactivity and butting/biting in males).

For the veterinary surgeon, intervention may be needed if one or more of these signs are also present: any other disease signs present – for example, nasal discharge; lethargy; concurrent weight loss; failure to prehend food after taking an interest; or not eating for over 7 days, especially in the post-hibernation period.

Anorexia frequently occurs post-hibernation and the phrase post-hibernation anorexia (PHA) has been coined, implying that this is a separate condition.

This is not the case: PHA is simply anorexia occurring in the period immediately post-hibernation. It should be investigated and treated as per anorexia at any other stage of the year – the causes are much the same.

Why does it occur so frequently post-hibernation? This is a stressful period in the annual cycle, in which the animal's metabolism is required to change dramatically. If current husbandry conditions, or if the hibernation conditions, were not adequate, then body stores are used up – this is especially the case where poor husbandry may result, over several years, in a cumulative effect.

The result is more correctly termed 'depletion', where the tortoise simply is depleted in terms of energy stores and metabolic resources to make the required step up in metabolism. Not only can this have a direct effect, but there can also be concurrent immune compromise, subclinical hepatic lipidosis, or dehydration resulting in renal failure.

Blood sampling (see Chapter 9.1) may show evidence of dehydration (raised urea and/or uric acid), lowered cell counts, lowered protein levels, lowered blood glucose and raised beta-hydroxy butyrate (if ketotic).

*Essentials of Tortoise Medicine and Surgery*, First Edition. John Chitty and Aidan Raftery.
© 2013 John Chitty and Aidan Raftery. Published 2013 by John Wiley & Sons, Ltd.

## Prognostic indicators

Prognosis is affected by:

- Degree of weight/condition loss.
- Degree of dehydration – that is, if there are obvious physical signs of dehydration, then the prognosis is much poorer.

**NB** Skin tenting is not reliable in chelonia.

- The length of time of anorexia.
- The quality of the environment and the willingness of the owners to improve it.
- Failure to urinate, which is a poor sign.

## Differential diagnoses for anorexia

- Depletion (see above).
- Sub-optimal husbandry – especially environmental temperature (see Chapter 2.1).
- Any systemic infection or organ failure.
- Gut infections or stomatitis, though these are often also secondary to the major cause of anorexia.
- Upper respiratory infections – again, often secondary to the major cause of anorexia (see Chapter 23).
- Stress – from new tortoises or from over-vigorous males (see Chapter 1.5).
- Overgrown beak (see Chapter 5.3).
- Freezing during hibernation – temperatures below freezing during hibernation may cause crystallisation in the eyes or forebrain, resulting in reduced vision and/or smell (see Chapter 25).
- Blindness due to other causes – for example, cataract formation (see Chapter 25).
- Endoparasitism.
- Follicular stasis in females (see Chapter 16).

## Approach

1. History – in particular:
   a. Environmental temperatures; especially, night-time temperatures need checking, certainly if not providing supplemental heating at night or if using a tortoise 'table'.
   b. Recent hibernation history and conditions.
   c. Mixing with other tortoises.
   d. Recent medical history.
   e. Feeding history over previous year.
   f. Recent urination/defecation.
   g. Reaction to food:
      - Ability to sense food?
      - Interest in eating?

2.  Examination:
    a.  Assess the body condition. The Jackson's ratio has been used as guidance for medium-sized *Testudo graeca* and *T. hermanni*. However, this has now fallen out of favour, and it is better to rely on physical palpation of legs and coelom and assessment of fat pads in the pre-femoral fossa and on either side of the neck (see Chapter 4.2).
    b.  Mouth – signs of stomatitis.
    c.  Eyes – sunken (dehydration or emaciation – extreme). Also check for cataracts, keratitis and signs of cold damage (see Chapter 25).
    d.  Respiratory rate/effort.
    e.  Shell or skin lesions.
    f.  Discharges – nose, mouth or eyes.
3.  Sampling and ancillary testing:
    a.  Blood sample for haematology/biochemistry assessment:
        - hydration
        - assessment of electrolytes
        - glucose and beta-hydroxy butyrate
        - white cell responses
        - anaemia/protein loss
        - major organ failure – especially liver/kidney
        - prognostic indicators (see Chapter 9.1)

    b.  Faecal sample (see Chapter 9.3). If problematic, then bath twice daily to induce defecation:
        - Wet preparation examined within 20 minutes of collection. It is important to assess the numbers of trichomonads and ciliates (especially *Nyctothera*) (see Chapter 9.3), both in terms of absence or overgrowth, either of which can be significant.
        - Flotation – nematode eggs.

    c.  Radiography:
        - Survey radiographs of body – dorsoventral and horizontal beam lateral, to assess:
            o  lung fields
            o  gut motility
            o  the presence of eggs in females

    d.  Ultrasonography:
        - to assess the liver and reproductive tract (in females)
        - to assess the heart and thyroid gland

    e.  Endoscopy of the coelom, cloaca and mouth, and pharynx and lungs, as indicated by other results
4.  Therapy – treat as indicated by the results (see the relevant sections in this book).

Frequently, the results will indicate a depleted tortoise.

## Therapy of the depleted chelonian

- Husbandry:
  - Correct environmental temperatures (20–32 °C for Mediterranean species; slightly higher for sub-Saharan).
  - Provide full-spectrum ultraviolet light for 12 hours daily. If at all possible, individuals should be exposed to direct sunlight for short periods each day.
  - Dry dock semi-aquatic species and give access to clean water once daily for swimming and feeding.

NB These animals will require hospitalisation in appropriate conditions!

  - Husbandry is usually the root cause and returning the animal to sub-optimal conditions will not help. If suitable accommodation is not available, then referral to specialised centres is indicated.
- Rehydration – depending on the degree of dehydration (see Chapter 5.6):
  - Daily or twice-daily bathing in warm clean water. Electrolyte or glucose mixes (e.g. Reptoboost, Vetark, Winchester, UK) may be added. Bathing is essential in all cases as it will also stimulate urination/defecation.
  - Oral rehydration by tube-feeding.
  - Intra-/epicoelomic; intra-osseous (or intravenous) routes are available in severely dehydrated animals.
  - Feeding (see Chapter 5.4.1):
  - Favourite foods should be provided to stimulate the appetite.
  - Animals suspected as being blind or cold-damaged should be hand fed.
  - Tube feeding of, initially, simple carbohydrate mixes [e.g. Critical Care Formula (Vetark, Winchester, UK) or Liquid Lifeade (Norbrook, Carlisle, UK)], progressing to higher-fibre formulae in herbivores [e.g. Oxbow Fine Grind (Oxbow, Nebraska, USA) or Emeraid Herbivore (Lafeber, USA)] or specialist mixes for carnivorous species [e.g. Oxbow Carnivore Care (Oxbow, Nebraska, USA) or Emeraid Carnivore (Lafeber, USA)]. Cat foods are not appropriate in any species.
  - Recalcitrant individuals (especially Leopard tortoises or Sulcata) or those on long-term feeding should have an oesophagostomy tube placed to reduce handling stress.
- Antibiosis – if indicated by the blood results or by clinical signs (see Chapters 9.1 and 9.4).
- Barrier nursing – many of these tortoises will be immunocompromised and may be receptive to or be shedding respiratory pathogens.
- Deworming – as indicated by faecal screening, even if only low numbers of parasites are detected.
- Re-testing haematological and biochemical parameters (especially those used for assessment of dehydration: see Chapter 9.1) at intervals to assess the effect of therapy, especially if clinical progress is not as expected.

# 11 Diarrhoea

Diarrhoea is much more common in herbivorous terrestrial species than in carnivorous aquatic species.

Faecal consistency can vary considerably even in individuals; therefore, a thorough history (including dietary activity) is required to ascertain whether there is a problem. True diarrhoea can be a life-threatening condition.

## Differential diagnoses

- Imbalance of gut flora and/or fauna (especially following sudden dietary change) or use of antimicrobials, especially metronidazole (see Chapter 9.3).
- Infection:
  - parasitic –
    - nematodes (see Chapter 29)
    - Protozoal (especially overgrowth of trichomonads) –
  - bacterial – unusual
  - fungal – very rare
- Gut motility disorders (see Chapter 12)
- Ingestion of gut irritant (see Appendix 3)
- Foreign body

## Approach

1. History – especially:
   a. Environment.
   b. Time since purchase or mixing with other individuals.
   c. Feeding – activity, changes in feeding, feeds given and garden feeding.
   d. Recent medical history, including drug dosing.
2. Examination:
   a. Assess the body condition (see Chapter 4.2).
   b. Mucous membrane colour.
   c. Respiratory rate/effort.

*Essentials of Tortoise Medicine and Surgery*, First Edition. John Chitty and Aidan Raftery.
© 2013 John Chitty and Aidan Raftery. Published 2013 by John Wiley & Sons, Ltd.

3. Sampling and ancillary testing:
   a. Blood sample for haematology/biochemistry assessment (see Chapter 9.1):
      - Hydration
      - Assessment of electrolytes
      - White cell responses
      - Red cell parameters
      - Proteins
      - Major organ function
   b. Faecal sample (see Chapter 9.3). If problematic, then bath twice daily to induce defecation:
      - Wet preparation examined within 20 minutes of collection. It is important to assess the numbers of trichomonads and ciliates (especially *Nyctothera*).
      - Flotation – nematode eggs.
      - Bacteriological culture – this is only considered of value if a more 'pathogenic' species (e.g. *Salmonella* species) is found in monoculture.
      - If melaena is present or suspected, a faecal occult blood test can be performed. In carnivorous species, false positives are possible if they have been fed carcase.
   c. Radiographs – dorsoventral and lateral views of abdomen to assess gut motility in terms of gaseous distension. A barium study may be indicated if a gut foreign body is suspected.
   d. Ultrasound is useful if organ failure is indicated and to help identify ileus.
4. Therapy – treatment should be based on clinical results. *Remember that the presence of some trichomonads is normal in a faecal wet preparation.* Otherwise:
   a. Nematodes – oxfendazole/fenbendazole.

**NB** Some care is needed when using benzimidazoles (see Appendix 1).

   b. Bacterial infection – appropriate antibiosis.
   c. Absence of faecal protozoa – obtain fresh faeces from a healthy animal of the same species; tube feed daily until normal gut function is achieved.
   d. Overgrowth of trichomonads – single dose metronidazole.
   e. Gut motility disorder – metoclopramide (foregut) or cisapride (hind gut).
   f. Surgery is indicated if a foreign body is suspected.
   g. Gut coating agents – for example, sucralfate – are indicated if the history suggests a possible irritant ingestion (see Appendix 3) or blood is found in the faeces.
   h. Supportive care:
      - fluids – oral (and systemic if severely dehydrated) (see Chapter 5.6)
      - correction of environmental factors (see Chapter 2.1)
      - supportive feeding (and avoidance of soft fruits/concentrate foods, which may induce gassy fermentation) (see Chapter 5.4.1)

# 12 Dyspnoea

## 12.1 Respiratory Disease

A dyspnoeic chelonian will often hold its head up, gaping its mouth open. More obvious pumping of the legs may be seen, which helps the respiratory effort. The glottis is often seen to be continuously open and there may be abnormal sounds and discharges coming from it.

### Differential diagnosis of dyspnoea

- Pulmonary disease.
- Tracheal lesion or obstruction.
- Glottis lesion or obstruction.
- Oral lesions.
- Penetrating wounds through the carapace.
- Nasal lesions – however, they do not usually cause dyspnoea.
- Pathology of other structures that compromise respiration. Enlargement of structures in the coelomic cavity can elevate the pleuroperitoneal membrane reducing the lung volume. See coelomic cavity distension (below).
- Immunosuppression from unrelated causes – for example, an inappropriate environment will predispose to conditions causing dyspnoea.

### Aetiology

- Viral:
    - herpesvirus
    - iridovirus
    - virus X – this is believed to be a picornavirus
- Bacterial – many bacterial agents have been identified as pathogens of the chelonian lung. They are all regarded as opportunistic pathogens with the

*Essentials of Tortoise Medicine and Surgery*, First Edition. John Chitty and Aidan Raftery.
© 2013 John Chitty and Aidan Raftery. Published 2013 by John Wiley & Sons, Ltd.

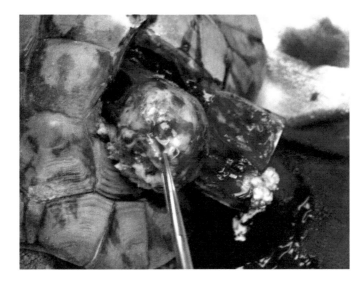

Figure 12.1.1    Removal of a pulmonary neoplasm via a carapacial flap.

possible exception of bacteria of the family Chlamydiacea, which can cause a systemic disease involving many areas of the body including the lungs.

- Parasitic:
  - o  protozoal – disseminated intranuclear coccidiosis is seen in several species
  - o  spirorchid flukes can cause a severe granulomatous reaction in the lungs of aquatic and semi-aquatic species
  - o  ascarid larva migrating can cause lesions in the lungs, which can lead to secondary bacterial pneumonia
- Traumatic:
  - o  penetrating wounds will predispose to a bacterial pneumonia
  - o  pulmonary haemorrhage secondary to trauma with no obvious changes to the carapace can lead to pneumonia, depending on the degree
- Inflammatory:
  - o  aspiration pneumonia
- Neoplastic:
  - o  fibromas and fibroadenomas are seen occasionally (see Figure 12.1)
- Toxic:
  - o  inhalation of irritants such as smoke is a common cause of dyspnoea
- Nutritional:
  - o  hypovitaminosis A is seen in aquatic and semi-aquatic species. The symptoms are associated with the squamous metaplasia and immunosuppression that it causes. Bilateral periorbital swellings are a more common sign; however, many develop secondary bacterial infections

## Diagnosis

- History.
- Clinical examination.

- Haematology.
- Biochemistry screen.
- Imaging – three radiographic views are necessary to evaluate the lung fields: the dorsoventral, lateral and craniocaudal views. The craniocaudal view is the best view to evaluate unilateral lung disease. Pneumonia in its early stages does not show up well on radiography. If it is easily visible, then the condition is advanced. A CT scan when available will provide a much more detailed image of the lung fields.
- Endoscopy – tracheoscopy is easy once the glottis is entered. A small 1–1.9 mm scope is needed, depending on the size of the animal. Visualisation of the lungs via the trachea is not possible in all species, due to the difficulty in descending the primary bronchi. An alternative route is via a small osteotomy in the carapace. This route is most useful in cases of focal lung disease, especially where the lesion is encapsulated, as the pathological tissues can be removed endoscopically (e.g. fungal granulomas) and treatment can be administered directly into the lesions (see Chapter 7.3). The pre-femoral approach can also be used, but repeat treatments via this route are more invasive. This approach can be difficult in focal lung disease: it is best reserved for diffuse lung disease.
- Pulmonary wash – hold the mouth open (sedation may be needed) and run a small flexible catheter down the trachea to the level of the lungs: a 1–1.7 mm diameter catheter, depending on the size of the animal. In the case of unilateral lung disease, it is difficult to control which lung is entered. Use dorsoventral radiographs to confirm that the catheter is in the correct lung. Slowly introduce 0.5–1.0% body weight of body temperature isotonic saline down the catheter. Gently rotate the animal around for a few seconds and then aspirate. Unfortunately, encapsulated lesions will give negative results with a pulmonary wash.
- Cytology – cytology can help evaluate the relevance of culture results and give an early indication of the possible diagnosis. A minimum of three smears should be prepared and air dried. Pathogens that fail to grow in culture media may be seen. Mycobacteria, parasitic and fungal organisms may be detected, which will help target further diagnostics.
- Culture and sensitivity testing – samples obtained from either a pulmonary wash, tracheal swab or endoscopically should be cultured for bacterial and fungal organisms as a routine.
- PCR – PCRs are available for several of the primary pathogens that can cause dyspnoea: herpesvirus, iridivirus, disseminated intranuclear coccidiosis, the Chlamydiacea group of bacteria and *Mycoplasma* species.

## Treatment

- Supportive care is essential for recovery. Optimum environment, rehydration, nutritional support and oxygen therapy will give the best chance of recovery.
- Antimicrobial treatment is best chosen by reference to a culture and sensitivity. Ceftazidime, enrofloxacin, marbofloxacin, doxycycline and amikacin are commonly indicated, depending on the target organism.
- Antiviral drugs have not been shown to be effective in chelonians; however, acyclovir doses of 80 mg/kg orally ranging from every 72 (Schumacher 1996) to

every 8 hours (McArthur *et al.* 2004) are quoted in the literature to treat herpesvirus infections. Due to the potential side effects, this should only be used in confirmed cases.

- There are many doses for antifungal drugs in the literature, but most have a very narrow therapeutic range, with frequent reports of serious side effects. Terbinafine appears to be relatively safe and so should be chosen when appropriate.
- Nebulisation therapy is commonly used. It will help by humidifying the airways. The aim is to get drugs directly to where the pathology is in greater concentration. There is controversy on how deep the nebulisation therapy can reach. Mucolytics such as acetyl cysteine or hypertonic saline are often nebulised together with the anti-bacterial drugs.

## References

McArthur, S., Wilkinson, R. & Meyer, J. (2004) *Medicine and Surgery of Tortoises and Turtles*. Blackwell, Oxford.

Schumacher, J. (1996) Viral diseases. In: *Reptile Medicine and Surgery* (ed. D.R. Mader), pp. 224–234. Saunders, St Louis, MO.

# 12.2 Coelomic Cavity Distension

The clinical signs of coelomic cavity distension are very similar to those of dyspnoea, being produced by dorsal displacement of the pseudo-diaphragm and restriction of the lung space.

Causes include the following:

- Ascites/peritonitis with fluid production – see Chapter 26 for investigation. Rarely, these will also present with fluid distension of the pre-femoral fossa.
- Perforating foreign bodies from the gastrointestinal tract. These form localised or even generalised abscessation of the related parts of the coelom and the lungs.
- Organomegaly – especially of the kidneys and liver.
- Gastrointestinal dilatation – 'bloat'. This may occur as a functional ileus, especially after radical changes in gastrointestinal fauna (e.g. after prolonged (> 1–2 days) metronidazole therapy or radical and sudden dietary changes, especially with the introduction of fermentable soft fruits to herbivore diets).
  - Diagnosis –
    - Radiography.
    - Endoscopy.
    - Cytology and culture of gastrointestinal contents – generally, these will need to be removed by gentle washing of the large intestine/cloaca by means of a soft rubber tube inserted per cloacum, followed by the introduction and withdrawal of warmed saline.

  - Therapy –
    - Identification and removal of the specific cause.
    - Therapy aimed against agents found overgrowing the gut. Due to gut immobility, these will often need to be given systemically or per cloacum.
    - Fluid therapy – systemic and oral.
    - Gut prokinetics –
      - metoclopramide
      - cisapride
    - The tube feeding of faeces from a healthy individual of the same species may help repopulate the gut with its normal flora and fauna. However, it is difficult to evaluate when this is necessary and if it helps. There is only anecdotal evidence that probiotic products are helpful.
    - Toxin adsorbents – for example, cholestyramine gel.
    - Nutritional support with a high fibre preparation – for example, Herbivore Care (Oxbow).

# 13 Otitis Media/Aural Abscess

No external ear is present in chelonians. The tympanum is seen from the outside as a circular scale level with the skin behind the eye. The tympanic cavity is large, extending quite far caudally. It connects to the oropharynx via the auditory tube.

## Aetiology

- Aural abscesses are more common in semi-aquatic species. The squamous metaplasia of hypovitaminosis A may be the predominant predisposing factor in these species.
- Immunosuppression from a poor environment and diet with opportunistic pathogens of environmental origin.
- Ascending infections from the oropharynx via the auditory tube.
- Any pathology affecting the patency of the auditory canal.
- Chronic inflammation will lead to squamous metaplasia.

## Clinical signs

- Bilateral or unilateral distension of the tympanic scute.
- White pustular material may be visible in the oropharynx, especially if pressure is applied over the tympanic scutes (see Figure 13.1).

## Diagnosis

- Check for underlying factors – environment, diet and other disease or chronic stress factors, such as inappropriate social groupings.
- Full physical examination.
- Needle aspirate for cytology.
- Culture and sensitivity samples should be collected at this time or during the surgery. There is a normal bacterial flora of the tympanic cavity in Chelonia.
- A haematology and biochemistry screen to help identify underlying concurrent disease.

*Essentials of Tortoise Medicine and Surgery*, First Edition. John Chitty and Aidan Raftery.
© 2013 John Chitty and Aidan Raftery. Published 2013 by John Wiley & Sons, Ltd.

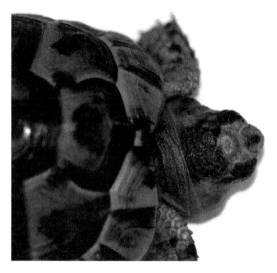

Figure 13.1    A bilateral ear abscess.

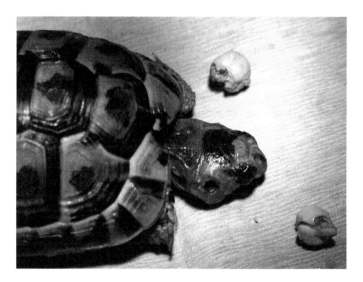

Figure 13.2    A bilateral ear abscess post surgery, with the pustular material that was removed.

## Treatment

- Surgery is needed – medical treatment will not cure this condition.
- Fenestrate the tympanum. Do not leave a ventral lip of tympanum, which would impede drainage. In general, it will be found to be much thicker in the terrestrial species than the aquatic species.
- Remove all the pustular material, which may come out in one piece, or it may be more friable and have to be flushed out (see Figure 13.2).

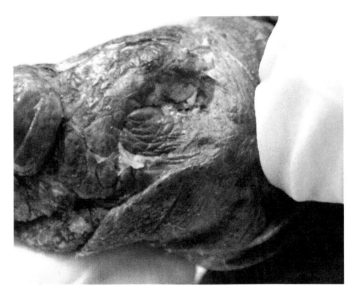

Figure 13.3   Chronically discharging ear infection, which will require flushing.

- Use a small intravenous cannula to flush the cavity with body temperature iso-tonic saline or dilute chlorhexidine (0.02% solution). Pay particular attention to ensuring that all the pustular material is removed from the caudal reaches of the cavity, and also the auditory tube.
- Use a local anaesthetic splash block for analgesia.
- Use non-steroidal anti-inflammatories to control inflammation and help with pain control.
- Antibiotic treatment based on culture and sensitivity.
- Some clinicians pack the cavity with an antimicrobial ointment or gel. Silver sulfadiazine cream is a common choice.
- Dry dock semi-aquatic species for 7–10 days after surgery (see Chapter 3.3.4).
- Flush the cavity daily until it remains clean, with no purulent discharge.
- The tympanum will heal by secondary intention. Some clinicians prefer to suture the tympanum (see Figure 13.3).

# 14 Egg Retention/Dystocia

## Normal oviposition

Most female tortoises need to be able to excavate a nest as deep as the length of their shell. They can be quite particular about the appropriate position and soil type. Others will just lay without digging a nest hole in their enclosure. Moving a female to an unfamiliar enclosure or providing a temporary nest box is more likely to be considered unsuitable by the animal. The Burmese mountain tortoise (*Manouria emys*) is an exception. The female constructs a nest by gathering sticks, dirt and leaf litter into a pile and then appears to take care of the nest for several days to weeks after oviposition.

Shelled eggs are normally held in the oviduct for variable lengths of time before oviposition, depending on the species: 1–2 months is common.

## Signs

There are no pathognomonic signs of egg binding. Animals may be clinically normal and the eggs found 'accidentally' during screening radiography. Clinical signs sometimes seen in conjunction with egg binding include the following:

- abnormal posture and gait
- posterior paresis
- anorexia
- lethargy
- restlessness
- tenesmus – occasional or prolonged
- cloacal discharge
- digging in several places

## Diagnosis

- Eggs may be palpable via the pre-femoral window. Place a finger on each side and gently rock the animal from side to side. Excess vigour may break eggs.

*Essentials of Tortoise Medicine and Surgery*, First Edition. John Chitty and Aidan Raftery.
© 2013 John Chitty and Aidan Raftery. Published 2013 by John Wiley & Sons, Ltd.

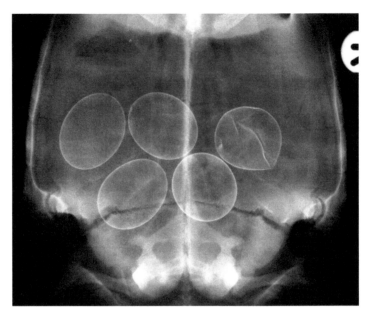

Figure 14.1    Egg retention with a cracked egg, which required a coelotomy.

- An egg may be palpated or visible per cloaca. Be careful not to push the egg into the bladder or faecal material through the pseudocervix.
- Radiography is the most important tool to diagnose egg binding. The number, size and shape can be evaluated. If greater than normal, the thickness of the shell may indicate that the egg has been present in the oviduct for longer than normal. Broken eggs will be seen, but whether they are adherent to the oviduct cannot be evaluated. Abnormally shaped eggs or broken eggs should be evaluated as to their likelihood to pass (see Figure 14.1).
- Ultrasound should be able to confirm whether there are any eggs in the bladder. Radiography is more reliable in determining the size and shape of the eggs, and whether they are likely to pass through the pelvis. It is also radiography rather than ultrasound that will identify broken eggs.
- Identifying the presence of large, broken or deformed eggs is an indication for surgery. Occasionally, they can be removed endoscopically. Check for environment, diet, previous medical history and social structure for underlying stress or disease factors.
- Full physical examination.
- Biochemistry and haematology screen. Phosphorus and total calcium levels are normally raised. Ionised calcium may be reduced, making supplementation an important part of the treatment (see Chapter 9.1).
- If the animal is otherwise in good health, provide the appropriate environment and a suitable nesting area. If the eggs are not produced in 10–14 days, then initiate medical treatment.

## Treatment

- Supportive care is essential. Ensure normal hydration status.
- Calcium orally every 12 hours at 400 mg calcium borogluconate per kilogram. If necessary, calcium gluconate may be given IM/IV at 50–100 mg/kg.
- Propranolol at 1 mg/kg orally once or atenolol at 7 mg/kg orally once. Beta-adrenergic blockers have been shown to potentiate the effect of oxytocin.
- Oxytocin is given at 5 IU/kg every 3–12 hours after the beta-blocker has been given and the oral calcium has started. If eggs are being produced at a rate of one or two a day, then continue until they have all being laid. If there is no response, then stop the treatment after 2 days. Surgical removal may be required.
- Ovariosalpingectomy is recommended over a salpingotomy to prevent recurrence of the problem.

# 15 Fallen in Pond

This is a common scenario for garden-kept tortoises in the summer, especially active wandering males.

The tortoise may be discovered after a varying amount of time, yet drowning is extremely rare even after several hours (or even overnight in some cases) submerged. Therefore, even if unresponsive, the tortoise should be thoroughly checked for signs of life (see Chapter 5.9). This high survival rate is essentially due to the tortoise's ability to lower its metabolic rate, to its very slow respiration rate and to its ability to withstand hypoxia.

The most common sequel is pneumonia due to inhalation of pond water.

## Diagnosis

Diagnosis is based on history. Most are presented apparently normal, so there are no obvious differentials.

## Therapy

In the acute presentation, the animal may be very weak and water may be draining from the mouth and nose. In these cases (if the animal is weak enough), a catheter may be inserted via the trachea and water aspirated in a similar manner to obtaining a lung wash (see Chapter 5.7). The animal should be warmed and may be placed in an oxygen tent if cyanotic. If collapsed and unresponsive, an endotracheal tube may be placed and the animal ventilated with oxygen (see Chapter 6).

The following should be given to all cases, even if presented apparently normal:

- Fluids – oral, intracoelomic or intra-osseous, depending on the state of collapse in which the tortoise is presented.
- Antibiosis – broad spectrum, such as ceftazidime, for 5–7 days as a minimum.
- NSAID – for example, meloxicam or carprofen for 1–3 days.
- Diuresis – furosemide is recommended by some authors, although the clinical effect is not clear. This drug should only be used in conjunction with fluid therapy. Use for a maximum of 2 days.

*Essentials of Tortoise Medicine and Surgery*, First Edition. John Chitty and Aidan Raftery.
© 2013 John Chitty and Aidan Raftery. Published 2013 by John Wiley & Sons, Ltd.

## Ancillary testing

### Haematology and serum biochemistry

In the acute case, this is unnecessary unless the tortoise is debilitated, in which case assessment of glucose, PCV, urea and electrolytes is essential to direct fluid therapy.

### Radiography

Radiography of the lung fields is of little value in the acute case, as lung changes are unlikely to be visible. However, horizontal beam assessment of lung fields should be carried out for animals unresponsive to therapy or showing signs of increased respiratory rate, effort or cyanosis after 7–10 days' therapy. Thereafter, treat as per chronic pneumonia cases (see Chapter 12).

NB Prevention is by preventing access to ponds.

# 16 Follicular Stasis

Follicular stasis refers to the condition where follicles are retained in the ovaries and do not progress to ovulation or undergo atresia. It may also be referred to as pre-ovulatory ova stasis. Accumulation of follicles can result in anorexia (see Chapter 10) due to the following:

- The space-occupying effect – in some cases, the ovaries can account for up to 10–15% of bodyweight.
- Circulating lipid and protein may suppress appetite centres. With ongoing signals to produce further follicles levels of protein, lipid and protein-bound calcium for production of eggs are at high levels. Hyperoestrogenism has been proposed as a possible mechanism, with resultant hepatic lipidosis and bone marrow suppression (Jones 2011).
- Depletion (see Chapter 10 for definition) – with ongoing egg production, depletion of body stores may occur, especially where husbandry is inadequate.
- Infection – ovarian necrosis is evident in some cases.

Follicular stasis should be included as a differential diagnosis for all anorexic female chelonians. The UK Mediterranean tortoises, particularly those of the Spur-thighed, Marginated and Hermann's groups, which have a reproductive cycle based on annual temperature variations, are commonly affected.

In these species, the reproductive cycle follows an annual cycle:

- Spring – rising temperatures induce vitellogenesis with formation and growth of follicles. These reach maximal size at the end of spring, when ovulation should be naturally induced (see below) and eggs laid.
- Summer – steady high temperatures induce cessation of ovarian activity.
- Autumn – falling temperatures induce ovarian activity, with small follicles being produced.
- Winter – low temperatures and hibernation, when ovarian activity is halted.

In the UK, these conditions and patterns are rarely achieved. Traditional methods of keeping tortoises at environmental temperatures result in continual fluctuations through the year, with few periods of consistent heat or cold. The result is that with

*Essentials of Tortoise Medicine and Surgery*, First Edition. John Chitty and Aidan Raftery.
© 2013 John Chitty and Aidan Raftery. Published 2013 by John Wiley & Sons, Ltd.

each temperature rise, follicle formation is stimulated, while periods of steady heat required for ovulation and egg laying rarely occur.

One of the few times for a temperature rise followed by a prolonged period of hot weather is in autumn, during the 'Indian summers' that occur every few years in September/October. This may result in ovulation, so shelled eggs are frequently found in female tortoises at pre-hibernation checks in these years.

The problem is exacerbated in lone female tortoises where there is no exposure to male pheromone or to their butting (Spur-thighed) or biting (Marginated and Hermann's), which seem to assist in stimulating ovulation. In other species, it has also been proposed that this state is reached due to inadequate environmental and pheromonal/physical cues for ovulation to occur. Failure to ovulate results in failure to form a corpus luteum and, hence, no stimulation for atresia of other follicles.

## Diagnosis

The following may indicate the presence of many large follicles on the ovaries:

- Ultrasound (Chapter 7.2) – non-invasive and capable of providing information regarding the size and number of follicles, as well as detecting evidence of follicular atresia (see Figure 16.1).
- Coelioscopy (Chapter 7.3) – invasive and requires anaesthesia. However, it enables much better visualisation of ovaries and other internal organs (e.g. liver and kidneys) and is the best means of diagnosing ovarian necrosis (see Figures 16.2 and 16.3).

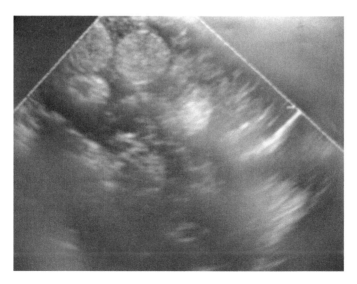

Figure 16.1   An ultrasound scan, showing multiple large follicles.

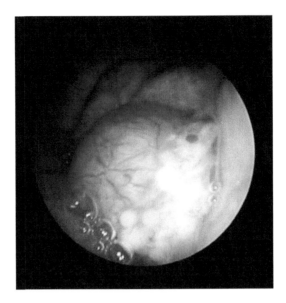

Figure 16.2   Follicles viewed by coelioscopy.

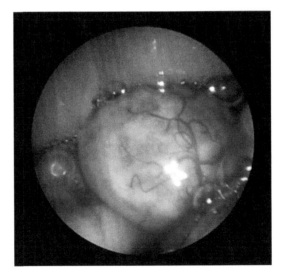

Figure 16.3   As for Figure 16.2, showing a follicle in the early stages of necrosis.

Blood biochemistries (see Chapter 9.1) may reveal a typical reproductive pattern with raised:

- ALT
- ALKP
- CK

- protein parameters
- total calcium/phosphate

**NB** Calcium and phosphate raised in the correct ratio of 1.5:1 to 2:1.

- triglycerides/cholesterol

In clinical cases of follicular stasis, the bloods may also show signs of dehydration, depletion and/or lympho-/leucopaenia.

If the female tortoise is anorexic or unwell, then the above findings confirming reproductive activity will raise suspicion of follicular stasis. However, a functioning female reproductive system may be coincidental rather than causative (especially when clinical signs occur at the relevant time of year). Therefore, follicular stasis can only be confirmed with sequential ultrasound or coeloscopy, confirming non-progression of vitellogenesis over a minimum of 2–4 weeks.

## Therapy

- Husbandry – in cases *where the animal is clinically well* and follicular stasis has been diagnosed on routine screening ultrasonography, changes in husbandry may be attempted. For Mediterranean tortoises in the UK, this may involve the following:
  - Short controlled hibernation at 5–8 °C, followed by environment controlled at 25–32 °C.
  - Introduction of a male tortoise of the same species. This animal should be from a known source and show no signs of infectious disease (if necessary, chelonid herpesvirus and *Mycoplasma* screening should be carried out: see Chapter 9.4). The male should be quarantined for 6–8 weeks prior to introduction to the female. Care must be taken to ensure that damage does not occur to the female from an over-amorous male – if this is a concern, then the tortoises should be maintained separately in the same room and only kept together for short supervised periods each day.
  - The female should be scanned every 2–4 weeks after mixing to monitor progress of the follicles for a period of 2–3 months.

In other species, return to conditions optimal to that species at its normal reproductive time (along with the introduction of a male) may also achieve an effect.

- Medical – various hormonal regimes have been suggested, though with little success. Proligestone has been proposed at 20 mg/kg, with mixed results. In our experience it has been ineffective, although this may be because it is only effective in the earlier stages of disease (progesterone is proposed as the major hormone-inducing negative feedback on release of gonadal trophic hormones from the pituitary: Jones 2011). When using proligestone, liver function should also be monitored, as hepatic lipidosis may be exacerbated. More recently, the use of deslorelin implants has been proposed; however, the role of gonadotrophin-releasing hormone (GnRH) is unclear in reptiles (Jones 2011) and there have been no controlled studies or anecdotal reports indicating a consistent response.

- Surgical – where follicular stasis is diagnosed, ovariectomy is the most frequent therapy. Depleted and clinically sick tortoises will require a period of pre-surgical preparation to ensure rehydration and adequate nutritional state. Plastronotomy is required for full exposure/access to the enlarged ovaries. Hysterectomy is not required unless there is concurrent uterine disease. This approach has the additional benefit for owners of lone female tortoises that the reproductive function is removed, thus preventing future relapses (see Chapter 8.3.2).

## Prevention

- Optimal husbandry.
- The presence of a male at the relevant time of year: regular ultrasonography to detect the increase in follicular numbers such that ovariectomy or husbandry changes may be performed before clinical illness.

NB If a lone female is scanned and shows no evidence of follicular activity, then introducing a male may stimulate ovarian activity – potentially leading to future problems.

## Reference

Jones, S.M. (2011) Hormonal regulation of ovarian function in reptiles. In: *Hormones and Reproduction of Vertebrates*, Vol. 3, *Reptiles* (eds D.O. Norris & C.H. Lopez). Elsevier, Amsterdam.

# 17 Orthopaedics

There is great diversity in shape and structure of bones among the varying groups of Chelonia. Dealing with orthopaedic conditions of reptiles requires knowledge of husbandry and medicine, along with the skills of an orthopaedic surgeon, to be able to diagnose and successfully deal with orthopaedic pathology. Often, a team approach is needed between the surgeon and the clinician. Most of the techniques used have come from mammalian medicine and are modified for the anatomical and physiological differences in reptiles.

## Evaluation of the patient

Prior to any decisions being taken on the management of an orthopaedic problem, the patient should be evaluated fully, to identify any concurrent or predisposing problems. This will allow a treatment plan to be formulated with investigations and treatments prioritised in the best interests of the patient.

A review of the husbandry is best undertaken before the clinical examination and should cover the following:

- Lighting – photoperiod, UV provision if required, position, life expectancy of UV source.
- Thermal provision – heat sources, thermal gradient achieved, reliability of the client's temperature readings, water temperature, night-time temperature, reliability of any temperature control system, ambient temperature and the possibility of unplanned temperature spikes.
- Humidity – hydrometer readings, means of generating humidity, water temperature, ventilation provided.
- Enclosure – type, terrestrial, semi-aquatic and so on, size, construction material, new or second-hand.
- Furnishings – substrate; hides; plants, live or artificial.
- Hygiene – frequency and method of cleaning, disinfectants used.
- Nutrition – food provided versus food consumed, feeding frequency, supplements given, water provision).

*Essentials of Tortoise Medicine and Surgery*, First Edition. John Chitty and Aidan Raftery.
© 2013 John Chitty and Aidan Raftery. Published 2013 by John Wiley & Sons, Ltd.

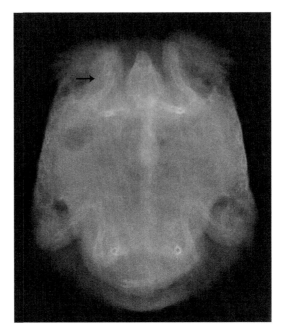

Figure 17.1    Fracture of the left humerus midshaft.

- Contact animals – in-contact animals, including those in the same premises, social structure, breeding history and quarantine protocols.

Previous medical history for the animal and any in-contact animals needs to be acquired and evaluated.

Full clinical examination (see Chapter 4.2) to attempt to identify the full extent of any problems and to provide information for the formulation of an effective treatment plan.

The clinician must be familiar with the species; otherwise, normal species variations may be misidentified as pathological changes. The shell of the Pancake tortoise, *Malacochersus tornieri*, for example, normally has a flexible and flattened shell, which has been misidentified as a symptom of a severe metabolic bone disease.

The minimum database for investigation of orthopaedic disease is as follows:

- Differential white cell count, packed cell volume and smear evaluation of cell morphology.
- Biochemistry panel, which includes creatine kinase, alkaline phosphatase, aspartate aminotransferase, cholesterol, calcium total and ionised calcium, uric acid, glucose, phosphate, total protein, sodium, potassium, chloride and urea in some species.
- Faecal parasite evaluation where indicated by species or history.
- Radiography – most reptiles presented are small enough to radiographically evaluate the entire skeletal system with two exposures (see Figure 17.1).

The aim is to identify if there is any predisposing or concurrent pathology that will affect treatment.

Radiography is an essential tool in orthopaedics to assess the extent of disease and/ or injury of the skeletal system. High-quality radiographs are essential, especially for the smaller patients that may also have decreased bone density adding to the difficulty in obtaining diagnostic radiographs. Digital radiography has greatly increased the value of radiographs, especially in the smaller patients, with its ability to improve image quality by reducing noise, removing technical artefacts and optimising contrast. Additionally, image manipulation enables proper evaluation of bone and soft tissue on the same plate without two exposures.

The skeletal system is assessed for any changes that could be associated with one of the metabolic bone diseases:

- generalised decreased bone density
- cortical thinning of the long bones
- pathological fractures, both old healed and recent
- angular deformities of the long bones
- deformities of the carapace, plastron and their joining bridges
- the opacity of the bones of the pectoral and pelvic girdles

## Supportive care

- Concurrent disease processes identified need to be treated.
- Environmental inadequacies need to be corrected.
- Fluid therapy.
- Nutritional support should be provided.

Solely concentrating on the orthopaedic problem is most likely to result in treatment failure.

## Healing of reptile bones

- Full clinical union takes approximately 50% longer than in mammals.
- Large cartilaginous callus is formed quickly, giving early stability.
- Radiography can be confusing in the first few weeks, as the large cartilaginous callus gives the appearance of a non-union.
- Time to stability at the fracture site is comparable to that for mammals.
- Environmental temperature, body condition and concurrent disease all have a dramatic effect on fracture healing.

## Initial fracture management

- If possible, splint unstable fractures and luxations as soon as possible. See bandaging techniques later.
- Fractures are painful, so start an analgesic programme immediately.

- Open wounds will be contaminated and antimicrobial therapy should be initiated immediately.
- Wounds should be debrided and irrigated as soon as possible.
- The animal's enclosure should be adjusted to prevent any activity that might result in further injury.

## Analgesic plan

Analgesia must not be ignored even if the animal does not appear to be in pain. A combination of an opoid, a non-steroidal anti-inflammatory drug and local anaesthetic blocks will provide balanced analgesia, allowing the lower end of the dosage range of each drug to be used and thereby reducing the risk of side effects such as respiratory depression:

- Morphine: 0.05–4 mg/kg intramuscularly (IM), subcutaneously (SC) every 12 hours.
- Buprenorphine: 0.02–0.2 IM every 12–24 hours.
- Meloxicam: 0.1 to 0.2 mg/kg IM or IV every 24–48 hours.
- Lidocaine 2% (2 mg/kg) mixed with bupivacaine 0.25% (1 mg/kg) diluted with sterile water for injection for more accurate dosing of smaller animals is a combination that we use. This is applied as a splash block directly on wounds or during surgery at the fracture site and as an incisional block. There are no reptile trials: the dose has been extrapolated from mammalian medicine.

## Surgical approach

Familiarity with the surgical anatomy is important for a successful outcome. Tissue handling should be as atraumatic as possible. The incision of muscles and tendons should be avoided; approaches separating muscles and tendons are preferable. The approaches used in reptiles are mostly modifications of the approaches used in mammals. Anatomy guides are not readily available and do not cover all of the species commonly seen. Whenever possible, surgical approaches should be practiced on cadavers. It needs to be remembered that following trauma, the normal anatomy is often disturbed, with surgical landmarks being unidentifiable. The *Biology of the Reptilia* series is the most comprehensive reference, but some of the titles are difficult to acquire. Another useful reference is Wyneken (2001).

These texts, in combination with an atlas of surgical approaches to the dog and cat, facilitate planning the best surgical approach in most cases. However, cross-species assumptions often have to be made about the anatomy. It should be remembered that the sprawling posture of most reptiles, where the body is slung between laterally projecting limbs, dictates different mechanically advantageous positions for external fixation devices and bone plates than would be used in mammals, with their erect posture.

# Fractures

Fracture reduction and stabilisation to facilitate healing can be just restriction of movement, external coaptation, external fixation, internal fixation or a combination. Decisions on the best treatment plan are best based on:

- the character of the species
- the bone affected
- the fracture site and type
- the age of the animal
- any concurrent disease

## Non-surgical management of fractures

Many fractures are held in a physiologically normal position by muscles and tendons. Many of these will heal in a functional position, with no interference except restriction of movement. During the early healing phase, simply restrict movement. Sometimes the bone density is such that even the application of a supporting bandage may result in further fractures. In these cases, the only option is conservative management with regular monitoring to identify any developing angular deformity early.

## External coaptation

- The use of bandages and other external splints and casts is common in reptile orthopaedics; however, they are not suitable in most chelonians, where attempting to retract the limb would put excessive pressure on the splint.
- They can be used in individuals with very deformed shells, where there is no effective fossa into which the limb can be withdrawn.
- The best results are obtained when it is used in simple, minimally displaced fractures.
- External coaptation can also be a temporary measure to immobilise the fracture while the animal is being stabilised and waiting for surgery.
- Often, this is the most suitable technique when bone density is too low to support implants.
- Cohesive bandages are the most common bandage type used for splinting in reptiles. They stick to themselves and not to the skin.
- Items such as tongue depressors, to increase stability, or extra padding materials, for comfort, can be incorporated in the layers.
- It is important to apply a bandage properly to avoid cutting off the circulation.
- Lay it on with mild constant unwind tension, to provide light compression.
- Monitor for any slippage that may cause constriction or failure of effective support.
- For greater strength in larger animals, the thermo-plastic polymers can be used to fashion casts. These materials are supplied in sheets that, when heated,

become malleable and can be moulded into the required shape of cast. They provide very strong, lightweight and water-resistant casts.

- Padding can be added with the thermo-plastic polymers to areas where there is the most pressure, to help protect the skin and underlying soft tissues.
- Cohesive bandages are usually used to hold the moulded splints in place.
- The principles of using casts and splints in reptiles are broadly similar to their use in mammals.
- The joints above and below the fracture need to be incorporated unless there is considerable intrinsic stability at the fracture site.

*Minimally displaced long bone fractures* can often be effectively managed by strapping the limb into the pre-femoral or cervicobrachial fossae. Check the fracture radiographically to ensure that it is anatomically reduced once it is strapped in position.

*Immature animals* that are growing rapidly should not have their joints immobilised. If their growth rate is slow, then if necessary joints can be immobilised in a physiological position, but this should only be for a short period. The more rapidly growing, the more the risk of joint deformities as a result of immobilisation.

*Fractures of the digits* rarely need support in chelonians. They are most commonly recognised in aquatic and semi-aquatic species, often secondary to bite wounds. In this case, control of infection is the most important consideration.

Terrestrial species in general have very short toes with elephantine limbs. Fractures of the carpus/tarsal bones and distal to these rarely require treatment.

## Aftercare

- Owners should be given written instructions on monitoring and maintenance.
- Bandaging materials should always be kept clean and dry.
- Exercise should still be restricted, as increased exercise will increase the risk of slippage and other complications.
- Any abrasions, loosening or angular deformity of the splint, discharge or bad smell should be reported immediately.
- If the animal shows sudden signs of becoming more uncomfortable, it should be investigated.
- Swelling and colour change of skin and soft tissues are not as obvious in reptiles.
- When a colour change to the skin is recognised, it will have been devitalised for days.

## External fixation

External fixation is not so easy to use in chelonians where repeated attempts at retraction of the limb will cause failure of the fixator. External fixation is also difficult to manage in aquatic species unless they can easily be safely dry docked for the duration of healing. Poor bone density is another contraindication for external fixation.

External fixation can only be used in species with limited fossae or individuals with deformities of the plastron and carapace such that there is no fossa. Pins must correlate with size of the bone. Those pins with a positive profile threaded area usually are more mechanically stable in reptile bones. Ideally, the central area of the pin shaft is factory-roughened to enhance the interface between the acrylic frame and the pin.

## External fixation of long bones

External fixation has the following advantages:

- It is minimally invasive, with little disruption of the fragments, their soft tissue attachments and their blood supply.
- The number and position of pins can be varied to meet the requirements of the fracture.
- If there is loss of bone, stabilisation can still be achieved as the area is bridged and normal bone length can be maintained.
- If there is contamination at the fracture site, there will be no implant there providing tracts to potentiate the infection.
- External fixation facilitates a quick return to function, reducing the incidence of fracture disease.
- It allows normal joint movement and better, more rapid healing.

If the fracture can be aligned, then it may be possible to place the pins percutaneously, two in each fragment, and then fit a Penrose drain or equivalent over the pins in what will be the final position when aligned. The fragments are then aligned and the Penrose drain filled with polymethyl methacrylate to set the position. Sometimes it may be necessary to place a small pin or Kirschner wire in the intramedullary space to facilitate correct alignment; however, the small size and contorted shape makes placement difficult. The most common end result is a type 1 external fixator.

### Aftercare
- Owners should be given written instructions on monitoring and maintenance.
- The pin entry sites need to be cleaned daily.
- Exercise should still be restricted.
- Any abrasions, loosening or angular deformity of the splint, discharge or bad smell should be reported immediately.
- After 4 weeks, assess healing radiographically.
- Healing should allow removal of the external fixator on average between 8 and 12 weeks.

## Internal fixation

Internal fixation techniques are rarely indicated in chelonians due to the limitations of their anatomy. It is indicated where external coaptation or external fixation are less likely to be successful in unstable displaced fractures. Intra-medullary pinning is occasionally used in chelonians, sometimes tied into an external fixator. Careful planning prior to intramedullary pinning is important, as the anatomy may direct the pin into the joint or within range of causing nerve damage.

Bone plates provide rigid fixation; however, their weakness is to angular forces. The main disadvantage is the more extensive surgical exposure of the bone that is required. The surgical outcome in reptiles can be significantly enhanced by following a minimally invasive strategy. Chelonian skin is less flexible than mammalian skin, which can cause problems with skin closure. Also, depending on the species, complex contouring may be needed to fit the plate to the bone. Bone plates are left permanently in position unless complications arise.

## Skull and mandible

- Skull and mandibular fractures are occasionally encountered.
- Trauma from being stood on or getting crushed by rocking chairs are common causes, closely followed by encounters with dogs.
- Iatrogenic fractures of the mandible can easily occur where there is pre-existing pathology during clinical examinations.
- Free-ranging chelonians are often presented with skull and mandibular fractures caused by encounters with road vehicles.
- Open fractures are more common in this site, with the increased risk of infection leading to malunion.

### Mandibular fractures

- External fixation is commonly used. Many small pins can be placed to stabilise many fragments. This allows feeding to continue while the fracture heals.
- Cerclage wiring can be used if there is just one fracture line, and a single oblique fracture line is the most appropriate fracture for this purpose.
- External coaptation can be an effective technique in some cases. It is the method of choice where bone density will not support external fixation pins. The mandible is stabilised by bandaging the mouth in a closed position and placing an oesophageal feeding tube for nutritional support until the dressing is removed. In severely displaced fractures, this may need to be supplemented by external fixation.
- Bone plating is contraindicated at this site in chelonians, due to the lack of enough soft tissues to close over the plate.

*Skull fractures* are best stabilised by bandaging the mouth in a closed position and placing an oesophageal feeding tube for nutritional support until the dressing is removed. Ensure that the oral cavity is clean and free of food before bandaging closed. Occasionally, wires may be used to stabilise unstable skull fractures.

## Amputation

Amputation is the treatment of last resort. Most chelonians do better without a chronically painful, non-functioning limb.

Indications are as follows:

- Where the pathology is so severe that it is most unlikely that alternative treatments will work.
- It is the primary treatment for severe limb trauma where there are tissue deficits incompatible with treatment; for example, where the distal limb has been eaten off by a dog or fox.
- Chronic septic synovitis with osteomyelitis.
- Locally invasive neoplasia.

The surgeon should follow the same surgical principles that are used in mammalian surgery. Radiographs are a very important part in the planning of the surgery. Often in cases of osteomyelitis, the pathology extends much further proximally than can be seen clinically.

Amputation is rarely an emergency procedure. The animal should be stabilised prior to surgery.

- Complications secondary to weight bearing on normal skin or bony prominences with little protective soft tissue are more likely in species with an average adult weight above 4 kg. The skin becomes devitalised and infection invades through into deeper tissues. In these animals, amputation of the entire limb at the shoulder or hip joint is recommended.
- In species with an adult weight below 4 kg, a lower amputation will provide a stump, which may help with ambulation.
- Healthy soft tissues should be used to help pad the bone stump.
- A flap of skin should be created such that the sutures are dorsally avoiding contact with the ground and the risk of contamination and breakdown.
- Bones can be sectioned or disarticulated.
- An osteotomy through one of the bones of the limb produces more granulation tissue, which better adheres the skin and soft tissues to the bone end.
- If disarticulating, then rongeur off the cartilage at the end of the bone. The theoretical advantage of removing the cartilage is that it will generate more granulation tissue, resulting in better healing.
- A local anaesthetic splash block can be used on transected nerves and other tissues as part of the analgesic plan.
- A small gliding prosthesis in the shape of a circular segment can be glued to the plastron just below the removed limb (see Figure 34.4), to prevent erosion of the shell and help with ambulation. Alternatively, a circular segment shape can be moulded from methyl methacrylate resin and attached to the same area. Adhesion is optimised if the area of plastron is clean and roughened where the prosthesis is to be applied.

- Some surgeons glue a small wheel to the plastron to assist in ambulation. However, these move well in one plane only and are more difficult to keep clean.

## Joint surgery

Chelonian coxofemoral joint luxation is the most commonly presented joint problem aside from septic arthritis. If presented early, they can be repositioned and then the limb bandaged in the pre-femoral fossa for 10–14 days to allow initial healing. Chronic luxations are more difficult to reposition. In some cases, excision of the femoral head is necessary.

The repair of an unstable stifle joint using an over the top technique modified from that described in mammals has been described in the literature (Hernandez-Divers 2002).

## Osteomyelitis

Osteomyelitis is common. It is most often a sequel to contaminated wounds.

Evaluation of osteomyelitis is based on the following:

- Visual appearance and palpation – swelling, heat and pain responses are not consistently present. Discharging sinus tracts are sometimes seen.
- Radiographic appearance – radiographically, osteomyelitis is seen as lytic lesions. The periosteal reaction seen in mammals is not present in Chelonia. Its radiographic appearance would be misidentified as neoplasia if using mammalian parameters of interpretation.
- CT scans are especially useful when the lesion is in the areas of the pectoral and pelvic girdles. These areas can be difficult to evaluate otherwise.
- Cytology can give an immediate guide as to what types of microbes are present. It is also useful to help interpret the culture. For example, if numerous Gram-negative rods were seen on cytology but only a Gram-positive cocci grew in the laboratory, then this may be a contaminant and not the main pathogen. Many pathogens are difficult to grow on normal culture media.
- Culture and sensitivity of samples, obtained by fine needle aspiration and surgical debridement.
- Blood culture – these are more commonly positive in chelonians than in mammals; however, there is an increased risk of contamination from the skin during venepuncture.
- Histopathology can help to differentiate infection from neoplasia or other resorptive diseases of bone.

### Treatment of osteomyelitis

- Surgical debridement and removal of all the necrotic infected material may be successful. Remove any bony sequestra or foreign material. These are often not seen radiographically.

- Amputation may be indicated depending on the extent and position of the osteomyelitis.
- Medical treatment with prolonged courses of antimicrobials based on culture and sensitivity. Both anaerobic and aerobic bacteria can be involved. Occasionally, fungal organisms have been isolated as the causative organism.
- Combinations of the above methodologies are most commonly employed.

## Reference

Hernandez-Divers, S. (2002) Diagnosis and repair of a stifle luxation in a Spur-thighed tortoise (*Testudo graeca*). *Journal of Zoo and Wildlife Medicine*, 33, 125–130.

## Further reading

*Biology of the Reptilia*, vols 1–22 (1969–2010). Edited Gans, with various individual volumes co-edited by A.d'A. Bellairs, T.S. Parsons, W.R. Dawson, D.W. Tinkle, K.A. Gans, R.G. Northcutt, P.S. Ulinski, F.H. Pough, F. Billett, P.F.A. Maderson, R.B. Huey, D. Crews, A.S. Gaunt, K. Adler and E.A. Liner. Academic Press, New York (1969–1982), John Wiley & Sons, New York (1985), Alan R. Liss, New York (1987), The University of Chicago Press, Chicago (1992) and the Society for the Study of Amphibians and Reptiles (1998–2010).

Wyneken, J. (2001) *The Anatomy of Sea Turtles*. US Department of Commerce NOAA Technical Memorandum, Miami, FL.

# 18 Fractures of the Shell

Shell fractures should be managed as an emergency. They can vary from simple cracks as a result of being dropped; smash injuries from encounters with lawnmowers or road vehicles where there may be missing pieces and extensive soft tissue damage; to crushing/grinding types of injuries caused by dogs. Fractures to the shell can result in the loss of body heat, fluids and the natural barrier against pathogens, and there often is extensive soft tissue damage, which may not initially be obvious (see Figure 18.1).

## Initial treatment

- Full clinical examination to evaluate the full extent of the injury and to reveal any other concurrent disease (see Figure 18.2).
- Provide analgesia – local splash block and parenteral, depending on the extent of the injury and the condition of the animal. Refer to pain management in Chapter 6.
- Anti-bacterial therapy is required, as these injuries are always contaminated.
- Non-steroidal anti-inflammatories to reduce the acute inflammatory response and also help with analgesia.
- Cleaning and irrigation of the wounds.
- Radiography – often, parts of the shell can be pushed into the body. Bite injuries can depress shards of shell bone into the underlying soft tissues. In fractures close to the spine, radiography will help evaluate tissue damage that may cause neurological deficits. Radiography may also reveal systemic disease, internal trauma and limb fractures.
- Apply wet to dry dressing and cover to protect the wound while the animal is stabilised (see Figure 18.3).
- Adhesive dressing tape can be used to temporarily stabilise the fracture. In simple, relatively stable fractures, this can be the only stabilisation necessary. If the lesions are judged very severe, make an early decision of referral or euthanasia (see Figure 18.4).

*Essentials of Tortoise Medicine and Surgery*, First Edition. John Chitty and Aidan Raftery.
© 2013 John Chitty and Aidan Raftery. Published 2013 by John Wiley & Sons, Ltd.

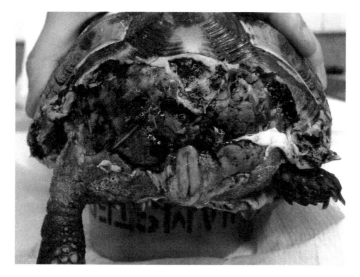

Figure 18.1    Shell trauma can require weeks of treatment.

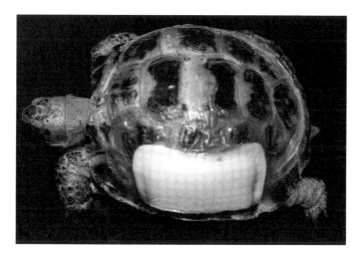

Figure 18.2    A protective dressing over a granulating shell deficit.

## Repair and wound management

- Debride the wound, removing debris and excising necrotic tissue. Depending on the severity, anything from just local anaesthetic up to a full general anaesthetic may be required.
- Lavage the wound with a large volume of warm isotonic fluid.
- Apply wet-to-dry dressing using isotonic saline or isotonic saline with 0.05% chlorexidine.
- Repeat the above three steps daily, or every 12 hours in very contaminated wounds.

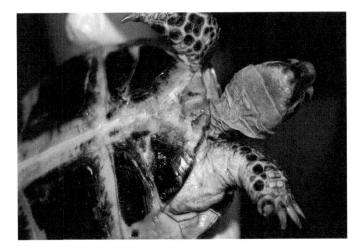

Figure 18.3   Penetrating wounds in the gular area can result in chronic infection of the bone marrow space.

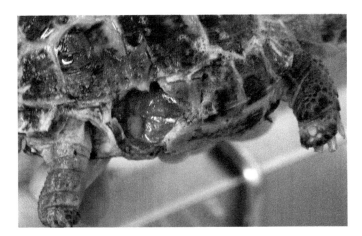

Figure 18.4   This animal healed after 7 weeks of wound management.

- Remove the dried-out dressing, without wetting, to aid in the debriding of the wound.
- The wound should look cleaner after each dressing change.
- Bleeding at dressing change is a sign that granulation tissue is starting to form, and the sign that it is time to change to a non-adherent, semi-occlusive dressing.
- If the coelomic membrane is lacerated, this needs to be sutured. Similarly, suturing is required if the lungs are exposed. Polyglecaprone 25 (Monocryl) and Polyglytone 6211 (Caprosyn) are examples of the most suitable suture materials. They are more rapidly absorbed and cause minimum inflammation and minimum tissue drag.
- In cases where there is a large deficit and suturing is difficult, products such as Vet BioSISt® (Cook Veterinary Products, Bloomington, IN) can be used to

provide a matrix for repair if there is no excessive exudation, bleeding or acute swelling, and if infection is under control.
- Fracture fixation requires a clean wound, which may take days to weeks to achieve.
- Continuing care of any exposed wound can be by use of:
  - saturated sugar solutions or honey
  - topical silver sulfadiazine ointment
  - hydrogels
  - alginates
  - polyurethane or silicone foams
  - collagens

All have their advocates and in an otherwise healthy animal with a non-infected wound all will result in good wound healing. Follow the principles of wound management used in mammals.

## Surgical repair of shell fractures

There are many different techniques of repairing fractures of the shell. Important considerations are as follows:

- Achieving stability.
- Starting with a clean, non-infected wound.
- Visibility – so that if infection starts, it will be seen and treated early.
- Elevate depressed fragments.
- Do not immobilise hinges on the plastron or carapace. This would include the caudal plastron hinge in *Testudo* species, which only give slight movement, to the plastron hinges of Box turtles and the carapacial hinges of the *Kinixys* species (the hinge-backs) (see Chapter 1).
- If the animal is not eating, place an oesophagostomy tube for long-term nutritional support.
- Fractures will take 1–2 years to heal.
- The fractures will be stable long before complete healing. In young growing animals, early removal of the fixation device will be necessary to prevent shell deformities.
- Do not allow hibernation until healed.
- Aquatic species may have to be dry docked for long periods (see Chapter 3.3.1).

## Screws and wire tension-band repair

- Screws are placed on either side of the fracture line.
- Orthopaedic wire is connected between the screws and tightened to apply compression across the fracture line.
- The best results are achieved if AO techniques are used to place the screws and the wire tightened to apply tension across the fracture.
- The fragments should be immediately stable.

- On removal, the screw holes will need to be protected while healing takes place. They can be covered with a protective bandage, which is changed every 5–7 days. Healing of the screw holes will take 4–8 weeks.

## Plates or metal bridges

- Curve the plate/metal strip to conform to the shell.
- Cut the metal bridge to a length 0.5 cm from the shell edge.
- Apply a bead of polymethyl methacrylate or epoxy resin 0.5 cm from the shell edge.
- Place the metal bridge ends in beads.
- Depending on the compression applied across the fracture line, orthopaedic screws may be needed.
- A high arch will allow wound management.
- Once healed, the retaining beads can be removed.

## Cable ties repair

- In this technique, the screws are replaced by saddle-type cable tie mounts, which are glued to the shell on either side of the fracture line.
- Cable ties are also known as zip ties or tie-wraps.
- A cable tie is secured on one side of the fracture line and then through a mount on the other side and tightened to provide compression across the fracture.
- A cable tie tensioning device can be employed to apply greater compression.
- Once healed, the cable tie mounts can be removed (see Figure 18.5).

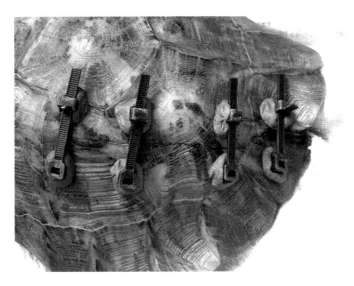

Figure 18.5    The cable tie repair of a fractured carapace.

## Negative-pressure wound therapy

Negative-pressure wound therapy, also known as vacuum-assisted closure, is especially well suited to the treatment of chelonians with shell damage where there is a deficit (see Lafortune *et al.* 2005).

## Polymethyl methacrylate (PMMA)

PMMA has a good degree of compatibility with body tissues and is used extensively in medicine. It has uses as bone cement in orthopaedics, it is a major part of dental composites and in many ocular prostheses, and it is also available as a glue to attach shoes to the hooves of cows. It is an excellent material to glue devices to the shell. It sets quickly, so the animal does not have to be restrained for long. In the past, it was used to bridge and stabilise fractures. This approach is now out of favour due to the risk of osteomyelitis developing out of sight. It is still often used to close the flap of a plastron osteotomy. Bridge any cracks before use to prevent the material filling the fissure, which would prevent healing. Mesh material will help the PMMA to bridge the crack rather than fill it. This method should only be used in non-contaminated surgical incisions.

Fiberglass and epoxy resins have been used in a similar way as PMMA.

## Reference

Lafortune, M., Wellehan, J., Heard, D., Rooney-DelPino, E., Fiorello, C. & Jacobson, E. (2005) Vacuum-assisted closure (turtle VAC) in the management of traumatic shell defects in chelonians. *Journal of Herpetological Medicine and Surgery*, **15**(4), 4–8.

# 19 Hepatic Lipidosis

While not a specific clinical sign or a single disease entity with clear signs resulting from it, hepatic lipidosis is very common in captive chelonians. It is implicated in many generalised disease states and frequently associated with nebulous clinical signs such as anorexia (Chapter 10) and lethargy (Chapter 21).

It may be seen as a primary or secondary disease, yet may also be present as a normal physiological state at certain times.

An excellent summary is provided by McArthur (2004).

Physiological hepatic lipidosis may be associated with hibernation and vitellogenesis and is associated with storage, mobilisation and utilisation of fat stores in these periods

However, hepatic lipidosis may also be associated with a pathological state and the following have been associated with inappropriate hepatic lipidosis:

- Inappropriate feeding of foods high in fat and simple carbohydrate, especially dog food, cat food and processed human foods, which may lead to obesity and hepatic lipidosis.
- Chronic hyperparathyroidism, whether nutritional-related or renal-related.
- Chronic hyperoestrogenism (e.g. follicular stasis: Figure 19.1) – see also Chapter 16 and Jones (2011).
- Hypothyroidism.
- Inappropriate hibernation in terms of both length and temperature.
- Chronic malnutrition.
- Inappropriate environmental temperature and/or light cycles stimulating lipid deposition pre-hibernation.

For a review of husbandry and diet, see Chapter 2.1.

As can be seen from this list of potential causes, there is no discrete boundary between physiological and pathological hepatic lipidosis, and the amount of fat present in the liver must be described in relation to the time of year, the animal's age and its sex, as well as simply the amount of fat seen in the organ.

*Essentials of Tortoise Medicine and Surgery*, First Edition. John Chitty and Aidan Raftery.
© 2013 John Chitty and Aidan Raftery. Published 2013 by John Wiley & Sons, Ltd.

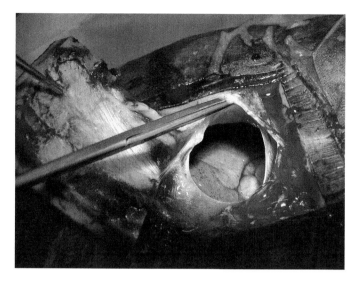

Figure 19.1    Fatty liver visible at coelotomy for follicular stasis.

Similarly, signs of hepatic lipidosis may not occur in isolation, but normally are in association with other disease states and, in particular, disease-causing anorexia. This is similar to the situation in other species, and the need for intervention and nutritional support must be assessed differently in obese animals compared to those in normal body condition.

## Clinical signs

- Anorexia (see Chapter 10).
- Lethargy (see Chapter 21).
- Biliverdinuria, though this is not consistent.

## Diagnosis

- History –especially in association with environmental, seasonal and reproductive factors described above.
- Examination – is the animal obese?
  - Is there evidence of follicular stasis? See Chapter 16.
  - Is there evidence of metabolic bone disease?
- Haematology/biochemistry (see Chapter 9.1).
  - Reduction in red/white cell counts.
  - Possible inflammatory changes in white cell counts (sometimes monocytosis, otherwise toxic changes) if secondary infection or if hepatic lipidosis is secondary to infectious disease.
  - Electrophoretogram changes – often elevations in the beta globulin region.
  - Reduction in albumin.

- o  Elevation in liver enzymes – though may often be non-specific (see Chapter 9.1).
  - o  Elevated bile acids (>80 mmol/l).
  - o  Elevated cholesterol.
  - o  Often elevated beta-hydroxy butyrate.
- Ultrasound – may show an enlarged liver with a homogenous appearance.
- MRI – may show liver enlargement.
- Coeloscopic appearance and biopsy – grossly appears with a distinct yellow colour. It may be friable on biopsy, so care is needed as excessive haemorrhage may result, especially if clotting factors are deficient in liver failure. Great care is needed to distinguish physiological hepatic lipidosis from pathological, and an experienced pathologist provided with a full clinical and husbandry history will be required to interpret such findings.

## Therapy

- Correction of underlying issues.
- Critical nutrition – the provision of a high-fibre, low-fat ration by stomach tube or oesophagostomy tube.
- Liver stimulants – for example, milk thistle extract (as medical-grade silybin – marketed for dogs/cats).
- Appetite stimulants – for example, anabolic steroids/B-vitamins.

## References

Jones, S.M. (2011) Hormonal regulation of ovarian function in reptiles. In: *Hormones and Reproduction of Vertebrates*, Vol. 3, *Reptiles* (eds D.O. Norris & K.H. Lopez). Elsevier, Amsterdam.

McArthur, S. (2004) Problem-solving approach to common diseases. In: *Medicine and Surgery of Tortoises and Turtles* (eds S. McArthur, R. Wilkinson & J. Meyer). Blackwell, Oxford.

# 20 Lameness

There is overlap between lameness, fractures and swelling. Reference may need to be made to Chapters 17 and 37.

## Investigation

- Environment and diet review. A complete review is essential, as a sub-optimal environment or diet can lead on to metabolic bone disease and/or a suppressed immune system, which predisposes to many of the causes of lameness listed below.
- Clinical examination of all body systems and areas is important, as an apparently unrelated disease process, which may be more important, can predispose to another condition causing lameness.
- A haematology and biochemistry screen will help to reveal underlying disease and give guidance on prognosis.
- Cytology of any lesions can often be diagnostic and will help to evaluate other diagnostics.
- Radiography is especially important for bone lesions.
- Culture and sensitivity of samples from lesions where pathogens may be present is especially important. Some pathogens are particularly difficult to treat – for example, mycobacteria and fungi – so identification is critical.
- Biopsy of a lesion is much more invasive than a fine needle aspirate, but it will give much more information, as the cell and tissue architecture is preserved.

## Aetiology

- Gout can manifest as the accumulation of uric acid crystals in joints. The distal limb joints are most commonly affected. The cause is most commonly chronic renal insufficiency and other factors such as dehydration, hypertension and cachexia predispose. Treatment is to prevent dehydration and if possible attend to the underlying condition. Gout is also often visceral, with gout crystals deposited over a variety of internal organs. Common sites are the pericardial sac, liver, kidneys, spleen and lungs.

*Essentials of Tortoise Medicine and Surgery*, First Edition. John Chitty and Aidan Raftery.
© 2013 John Chitty and Aidan Raftery. Published 2013 by John Wiley & Sons, Ltd.

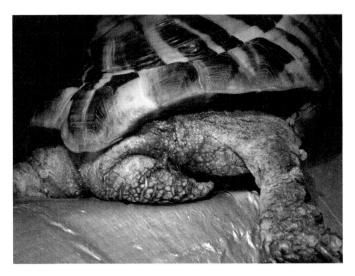

Figure 20.1    Femoral head ostectomy via the caudal approach.

- Synovitis. Inflammation of the synovial membranes is painful when the joint is moved. There is usually reluctance to move. It can be due to trauma, infection, ligament rupture or neoplasia. There is usually an accumulation of synovial fluid in the joint secondary to the inflamed synovium, which makes arthrocentesis easier. Cytology, culture and sensitivity of a synovial fluid sample are important in the formulation of a treatment plan.
- Neoplasia can cause lameness. The degree of lameness will depend on the tissue involved and on the type of neoplasia. It may be due to pain, lack of function or neurological damage, or a mix of all three. Cytology of a fine needle aspirate, biopsy and diagnostic imaging may all help with the diagnosis and prognosis.
- Luxation of any limb joint can be seen. These usually are diagnosed by radiography. Successful reduction of the luxation should be confirmed radiographically. If successfully reduced, then it can be effectively managed by strapping the limb into the pre-femoral or cervicobrachial fossae. Re-evaluate after 10–14 days by radiography and also gently manipulate the joint. Sedation is usually required to allow a diagnostic manipulation. If it is not stable, then a further 10–14 days of strapping in the fossa will be needed. Some cases will need surgical repair. The coxofemoral joint is the joint most commonly presented with a luxation in chelonians. If presented early, they can be repositioned and then the limb is bandaged in the pre-femoral fossa for 10–14 days to allow initial healing. Chronic luxations are more difficult to reposition. In some cases, excision of the femoral head is necessary (Figure 20.1: see also Raftery 2004).
- Developmental bone lesions include angular deformities of the bones, bone cyst formation and abnormal joint surfaces. These put abnormal pressures on the joints, tendon, ligaments and muscles. Movement and function of the limb may be abnormal and in the longer term these abnormalities lead to degenerative joint disease.

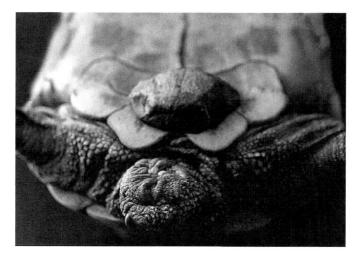

Figure 20.2    Sliding prosthesis to help locomotion.

- Degenerative joint disease is a common sequel of many chronic pathologies that affect the limb. The chronic use of NSAIDs has not been studied in Chelonia. Short courses to settle down flare-ups are most commonly used. A small gliding prosthesis in the shape of a circular segment can be glued to the plastron, just below the affected limb, to prevent erosion of the shell and help with ambulation. The circular segment shape can be moulded from methyl methacrylate resin or equivalent (see Figure 20.2).
- Fracture of a limb is a common cause of lameness. Radiography is required for diagnosis and to help formulate a treatment plan (see Chapter 17).
- Neurological disease:
  - ○ Spinal lesions can be caused by trauma, infection or neoplasia. Radiography is usually necessary for a diagnosis; however, CT and MRI will give more information.
  - ○ Central nervous system disease can cause abnormal gaits or just generalised weakness.
  - ○ Neurotoxins cause symptoms similar to those seen in mammals. The most commonly seen neurotoxins are insecticides used in horticulture, such as the organophosphates and the carbamates. Reptiles in general are more suspectible to the toxic effects of these compounds than mammals. Ivermectin is extremely toxic to Chelonia and causes a paresis or flaccid paralysis (see Appendix 3).
  - ○ Uroliths, egg binding and constipation can cause lameness by putting pressure on the nerves.
  - ○ Freeze damage has been reported as causing lameness/abnormal gait.
- Thiamin deficiency is seen in semi-aquatic and aquatic chelonians fed exclusively with a diet of defrosted fish. It results in muscle twitching and incoordination.
- Ligament rupture/avulsion as a cause of lameness is diagnosed by palpation, usually with the animal sedated. Radiography is important to rule out fractures and other bone lesions (see Hernandez-Divers 2002).

- Metabolic bone diseases such as secondary nutritional hyperparathyroidism cause lameness. The hypocalcaemia causes neuromuscular excitability with muscle tremors. Pathological fractures can also be seen, but are rare in chelonians compared to the incidence in other reptiles with metabolic bone disease of nutritional origin.
- Trauma is a common cause of lameness due to pain, damage to the limb or to the nerves going to the limb.
- Generalised weakness due to any cause.
- Hypothermia causes a generalised weakness and the animal can be in a state of torpor.
- A thermal injury such as a burn, either chemical or thermal, causes areas of tissue necrosis with associated inflammation, secondary infection, pain and lameness.
- Hypervitaminosis A is seen when excess vitamin A is administered parenterally. It causes sloughing of the soft skin, mainly on the legs, which is painful and results in lameness.

## References

Hernandez-Divers, S. (2002) Diagnosis and repair of a stifle luxation in a Spur-thighed tortoise (*Testudo graeca*). *Journal of Zoo and Wildlife Medicine*, 33, 125–130.

Raftery, A. (2004) In: *Medicine and Surgery of Tortoises and Turtles* (eds S. McArthur, E. Wilkinson & J. Meyer), p. 463. Blackwell, Oxford.

# 21 Lethargy

Lethargy is a common presentation in Chelonia.

However, it is an unusual sign on its own and is most commonly associated with anorexia (see Chapter 10) and/or weight loss or failure to grow.

For this reason, it is termed by some authors, ADR syndrome ('ain't doin' right'), as there is no single presenting sign, but rather a generalised malaise and failure to thrive.

The investigation for such a generalised sign is, accordingly, very general. The causes and investigation are extremely similar to those outlined in Chapter 10.

Triage of these cases is very important, as (in order of clinical urgency) lethargy may be due to the following causes:

- physiological – that is, 'normal'
- environment-driven
- illness
- debility/collapse

In particular, is the animal lethargic as part of a clinical condition? Patterns of activity are important, as chelonia are often inactive for large parts of the day. Older tortoises too may be become much less active. However, if 'normal' these animals may still be extremely active at certain times and will still have a good appetite. Semi-aquatic species are often extremely inactive, being 'lie in wait' hunters (see Chapter 1.5); however, they will usually become extremely active when disturbed/handled, and will usually feed readily. As in all clinical cases, it is important that an owner understands his or her own animal. Departures from an individual's normal behaviour may represent a disease state. Problems occur with new animals and inexperienced owners where the normal behaviour simply is not known. If in doubt, investigate as if the animal is unwell.

Environmental conditions are extremely important: in particular, temperatures should be noted (including water temperature in semi-aquatic species), as both low and high temperatures may lead to inactivity and lethargy. These investigations are

*Essentials of Tortoise Medicine and Surgery*, First Edition. John Chitty and Aidan Raftery.
© 2013 John Chitty and Aidan Raftery. Published 2013 by John Wiley & Sons, Ltd.

described in Chapter 2.1. It is particularly important to check these temperatures accurately – especially at night, when the ambient temperature in uninsulated vivaria or tables may fall.

Poor water quality may prevent semi-aquatic species from entering water. If land space in the vivarium is also restricted, they may show forced inactivity (see Chapter 2.1).

Social groups should be assessed – most species are not social, yet may be kept in groups in captivity. 'Bullying' may therefore occur, and less assertive or smaller individuals may be driven away from heat sources and food, and tend to hide (see Chapter 1.5).

## Clinical investigation

In general, if there is no abnormality found on clinical examination and the animal appears in good physical condition, with no obvious environmental concerns, then it is worth re-examining in 2–3 weeks to reassess weight and condition. Loss in either parameter or persistent lethargy should prompt a detailed diagnostic investigation. If taking this course, it is vital that there is good communication between veterinarian and owner, and that the owner understands that he or she should contact the veterinarian before 2–3 weeks should signs worsen or change. For the inexperienced clinician, this may also be a good time to consider consulting with or referring to a more experienced colleague.

The full clinical investigation (as mentioned earlier) should follow the same course as for the anorexic animal (see Chapter 10). However, the following tests should take increased priority in the lethargic animal:

- Horizontal beam radiography of lung fields should be performed (see Chapter 12). Chelonia with pneumonia will often lower the metabolic rate in order to cope with reduced oxygen exchange ability, shunning heat sources and becoming less active (see Chapter 1.5).
- In aged animals, it is important to thoroughly check joints and assess muscle tone and bulk. Osteoarthritis or gout may occur more frequently in these animals and pain can be a reason for inactivity.

# 22 Soft Tissue Masses

Soft tissue masses are a common presentation in captive Chelonia. Differential diagnoses are similar to those for the same presentation in other species, and to a large extent the clinical approach for a soft tissue mass in a tortoise is similar to that for a mass on a dog.

The following are the most likely differentials for a soft tissue mass:

- abscess or granuloma
  - bacterial
  - fungal
  - parasitic
  - mycobacterial
  - foreign body
- neoplasia – especially older individuals
- haematoma

As described above, the investigation can follow similar lines to those employed in other species.

## History

In particular, the following may be relevant:

- reported trauma
- recent acquisition or importation
- the presence of other stressors may be of importance

While husbandry is not always of direct cause (other than in aquatic species, where water-quality parameters are very important – see Chapter 2.1), it is vital for optimal recovery, especially after surgery.

*Essentials of Tortoise Medicine and Surgery*, First Edition. John Chitty and Aidan Raftery.
© 2013 John Chitty and Aidan Raftery. Published 2013 by John Wiley & Sons, Ltd.

## Clinical examination

As ever, a thorough clinical examination is important not just to attempt to evaluate the mass itself (with respect to size, degree of invasion of local tissues, appearance and likelihood of being able to completely excise), but also to identify other masses and any important underlying causes:
- Palpation – is the mass
  - o Solid?
  - o Fluid-filled/turgid?
  - o Does it appear to be connected to underlying structures?
  - o If so, how large does it appear?

## Clinical investigation

Where masses appear to be invading deeper structures, radiographs are useful to determine involvement of shell and/or bony structures. Horizontal beam lateral views of the lung fields may be useful before attempting excision of masses determined to be malignancies. Ultrasound may be useful to assess the size of masses, their invasiveness and their response to therapy. CT scans may be utilised if available to determine invasion into other tissues and metastases into internal soft tissues.

Biopsy is essential in such cases and a variety of techniques can be used (see Chapter 5.7):

- Fine-needle aspirate and cytology. Particularly appropriate for fluid-filled masses. Does not require anaesthesia/sedation, but will give limited information on solid masses as samples do not show tissue architecture.
- Impression smears – may be used for ulcerated masses. However, can be affected by surface contamination, so should be performed after scraping the surface.
- Trucut samples – very useful for large masses. In some cases, may be performed under local anaesthesia, but may require anaesthesia/sedation of the patient if biopsying masses that enter deeper body structures. In these cases, biopsy under ultrasonic guidance may help.
- Excision biopsies – either complete or partial (i.e. wedge biopsies). Appropriate for small skin masses or for very large lesions. Will require anaesthesia or sedation, but will give maximum information regarding the mass. As ever with biopsies, attempts must be made to include representative samples – if necessary, separate sections of superficial and deeper parts of the mass should be taken. Margins are also useful to determine invasiveness.

## Therapy

Obviously, this depends on diagnosis. In general, though, it is preferable to excise soft tissue masses. Where deep tissues or bones of one limb are affected by a granuloma or tumour, then amputation may be considered.

Where excision is not possible, palliative care may be possible by:

- debulking of tumours
- intra-lesional injections of appropriate antimicrobials alongside systemic anti-microbials in the case of granulomata
- supportive care and correction of underlying disease and husbandry defects
- marsupialisation of cavitated lesions, allowing regular access for packing and cleaning

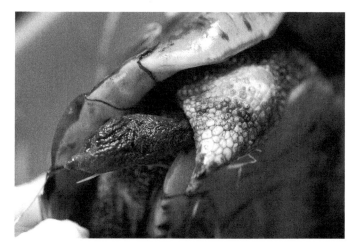

Figure 22.1    A prolapsed phallus in an aged Hermann's tortoise. Note the swelling on the caudal aspect of the tail. This represented a large sarcoma, invading the cloacal tissue. Prolapse was due to penetration of the mass into the spinal column and resultant paralysis. The tortoise was euthanased.

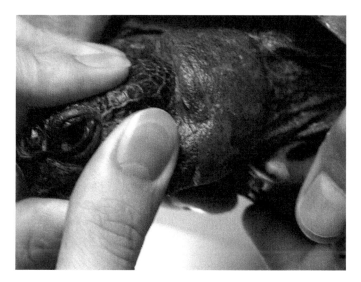

Figure 22.2    A diffuse mass on tortoise neck. Biopsy showed this to be a bacterial infection.

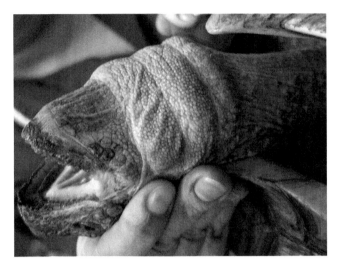

Figure 22.3   A diffuse mass on the ventral neck of a Sulcata. Biopsy showed this to be a mycobacterial infection and the animal was euthanased.

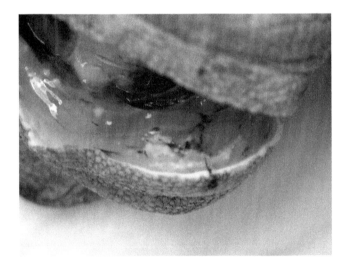

Figure 22.4   At post-mortem examination, the cut surface shows the typical granular appearance of a mycobacterial granuloma.

Euthanasia should be considered in the event of:

- underlying disease that is too severe and judged unlikely to respond to therapy
- invasive tumour or metastases with considerable invasion of underlying/ surrounding structures in an unwell animal
- zoonotic disease – for example, mycobacteriosis
- the cost of treatment is beyond the resources available – euthanasia is often a more humane option than no action

See Figures 22.1, 22.2, 22.3 and 22.4.

# 23 Nasal Discharge

## Clinical examination

- A full history should be obtained, followed by a complete clinical examination together with a review of the environment and diet.
- What type of discharge is present: serous, mucoid, purulent or blood? Is it copious or only occasional? Is it bilateral or unilateral, and is there any damage or erosion of the nares or surrounding tissues (see Figures 23.1 and 23.2)?
- Is a discharge visible at the choana?
- Oral lesions, ocular or any other signs related to upper respiratory tract disease should be recorded.
- Many pathogens that can cause an upper respiratory infection with a nasal discharge chronically infect individuals but only cause symptoms when there is a degree of immunosuppression caused another disease, environment, diet or inappropriate social groupings.

## Diagnostics

- Haematology and biochemistry screen will help to reveal underlying disease.
- Cytology can give rapid answers. Cytology will also help to evaluate the relevance of culture results, as many pathogens will not grow in culture media and may be seen on cytology. Fungal organisms may be seen, which would indicate need for a fungal culture.
- Culture and sensitivity testing is very important, as there are many possible opportunist pathogens that, if they become established, can be difficult to treat.
- PCRs are available for several of the primary pathogens that can cause a nasal discharge: *Mycoplasma* species, herpesviruses, Iridovirus and bacteria of the Chlamydiacea group. An oropharyngeal swab or a swab of the nasal discharge at the external nares can be collected using a micro-swab.
- Serology:
  - Serology is available for *Mycoplasma agassizii*, the most common chelonian species, but it may not detect exposure to other mycoplasmas. Serology is

*Essentials of Tortoise Medicine and Surgery*, First Edition. John Chitty and Aidan Raftery.
© 2013 John Chitty and Aidan Raftery. Published 2013 by John Wiley & Sons, Ltd.

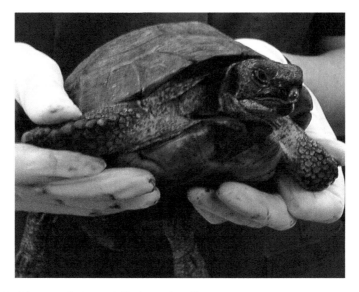

Figure 23.1    Mucopurulent nasal discharge in a *T. gracea*.

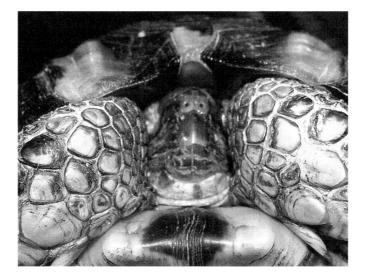

Figure 23.2    Serous nasal discharge.

regarded by some as the best test to screen healthy animals for mycoplasma. Culture is also available, but difficult (see Chapter 9.4).

- o Chelonian herpesvirus serology tests are available. However, seroconversion is slow. The test is influenced by the species of tortoise and the virus serotype. Latently infected animals often test negative.
- Imaging may be of use to assess whether there is also lower respiratory disease. Where they are available, CT scans give the most information. Radiography

is more common, with the skyline view (craniocaudal view) usually giving the most information.

- Endoscopy of the nasal cavities is limited, especially in the small to medium-sized tortoises. A needlescope (1.2 mm) can fit through the external nares of a 2–3 kg tortoise (depending on the species) and give a view of the nasal cavity. It is more likely to be diagnostic where the discharge is unilateral. It may have to be combined with a nasal wash so that any lesion can be visualised.
- Nasal wash – holding the animal's head towards the floor, instil about 0.5 ml of warm isotonic saline and collect samples for cytology either at the choana or from the fluid escaping from the external nares. Samples that are discharging naturally are usually more productive. The value of a nasal wash is to clear away discharges, collect diagnostic samples and permit better visibility of any lesion with rhinoscopy.

## Aetiology

- Mycoplasmas are a common cause of nasal discharge and have been isolated from many species of terrestrial chelonians. Subclinical infections are common, with convalescence and recrudescence of clinical signs. Culture is very difficult. Diagnosis is achieved with either serology or PCR. False negatives can occur and there are some strains that are not believed to cause clinical disease (see Chapter 9.4).
- Herpesvirus infection is a common cause of nasal discharge in terrestrial tortoises: rhinitis, conjunctivitis, stomatitis and glossitis. Herpesviruses can also affect the central nervous system, gastrointestinal tract, urinary tract, liver and spleen. There are many chelonian herpesviruses. Many species have been found to have their own endemic species of herpesvirus. Flare-ups of clinical signs can be associated with stress/concurrent infections/immunosuppression. More severe infections are seen when there is mixing of different species, allowing the herpesviruses to jump between species. PCR tests are the best diagnostic tools and can be used to differentiate between the different chelonian herpesviruses. Herpesviruses can be seen as intranuclear inclusions on cytology and histologically.
- Ranavirus infection has been associated with rhinitis and palpebral oedema. It has also been associated with pneumonia, ulcerative tracheitis and oesophagitis and a vasculitis in multiple organs. PCR tests are used for diagnosis. Histology will reveal intracytoplasmic inclusions, which can be evaluated by electron microscopy.
- Bacteria of the family Chlamydiacea are potential pathogens, causing respiratory disease with a nasal discharge. PCR is the best way to diagnose this organism, but speak to the laboratory first to check whether their PCR is appropriate.
- Fungal organisms are usually regarded as opportunistic pathogens. Often, they cause a unilateral nasal discharge. Diagnosis is by a combination of cytology and culture.
- Foreign bodies are not common. They are usually identified by rhinoscopy. A nasal flush may be able to dislodge them.
- Neoplasia is a very rare cause of nasal discharge in chelonians.

- Bacterial rhinitis caused by a range of opportunistic pathogens is common. The primary cause of the rhinitis is often not detectable. Many of these bacteria are normal inhabitants of the respiratory and gastrointestinal tract. Identify with culture and use the sensitivity as a guide to treatment, as innate resistance to many anti-bacterials is common.

## Treatment

- Environment and diet improvements are very important. Healthy tortoises can cope with sub-optimal conditions, but need optimum conditions to have the best chance of recovery.
- Concurrent disease needs to be treated. Several of the agents that cause nasal discharge in chelonians are present as latent or subclinical infections, and when other conditions occur they can become clinical.
- Systemic antimicrobials are required when a bacterial or fungal pathogen has been identified. When a viral agent has been found, concurrent opportunistic bacterial pathogens are also usually present, so antimicrobials are still indicated.
- Nebulisation of antimicrobial drugs and other agents to help clear mucus and to humidify the airways has been advocated. In chelonians, there is only anecdotal evidence of the efficiency of this method of administering medication. If used, it should be combined with systemic antimicrobials.
- Nasal flushing can be of value therapeutically by flushing out accumulated discharges. If collected, the fluid can be of diagnostic value. Use isotonic saline at between 30 and 37°C. Large volumes and repeat flushings over several days may sometimes be needed to dislodge stubborn deposits. Use a 22–24 gauge intravenous cannula introduced through the external nares to deliver the fluid. Both sides should be flushed.
- Antiviral agents – acyclovir has been used to treat symptoms associated with herpesvirus infections. There is no pharmacological data on the use of this drug in chelonians. However, it has been used, without apparent adverse effects, in several species at a range of doses. It will not eliminate the virus: any positive animal will be a carrier of that herpesvirus for life.

# 24 Ocular and Conjunctival/Palpebral Swelling

## Normal anatomy

- Eyelids well developed, with lower lid larger and more mobile.
- A nictitating membrane is present: it can make examination of the cornea difficult.
- The hardarian gland is present in the anterior portion of the bony orbit and it opens in the conjunctival sac through several ducts.
- The lacrimal gland is situated in the caudal aspect of the bony orbit. It also opens into the conjunctival sac through ducts.
- The nasolacrimal duct is believed to be absent in chelonians.

Investigation of ocular or periocular disease should start with a complete evaluation of the environment and diet and a complete clinical examination. A full history should be collected. Important points would include (see Figure 24.1):

- the history of contact with other tortoises in the past two years
- whether the lesion is uni- or bilateral
- if part of a group, whether several are affected
- whether the lesion is progressive

The ocular examination is covered in Chapter 25, which also covers conditions of the eyeball; that is, the cornea and the anterior and posterior segments of the eye.

Many of the possible pathogens that can cause ocular or periocular disease can be present as latent or subclinical infections, which become clinical when the animal is immunosuppressed by either non-ideal environmental conditions or a concurrent disease.

## Periocular, palpebral or ocular swelling differential list

- Herpesvirus infections of tortoises can cause ocular discharge with palpebral swelling, in addition to rhinitis and stomatitis.
- Ranaviruses of the family Iridoviridae can cause palpebral oedema in addition to rhinitis, ulcerative tracheitis, pneumonia, ulcerativitis pharyngitis and oesophagitis.

*Essentials of Tortoise Medicine and Surgery*, First Edition. John Chitty and Aidan Raftery.
© 2013 John Chitty and Aidan Raftery. Published 2013 by John Wiley & Sons, Ltd.

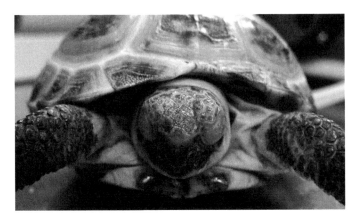

Figure 24.1    A palpebral oedema in a *T. horsfeldii* with underlying renal insufficiency.

- *Mycoplasma* spp. are common causes of rhinitis in tortoises, which is usually accompanied by ocular discharge, conjunctivitis and palpebral oedema.
- *Chlamydia* spp are commonly identified in tortoises with a nasal discharge. Blepharitis can also be present.
- *Pasteurella* spp. have been isolated from tortoises with ocular discharge, conjunctivitis and palpebral oedema. However, it can also be found in healthy individuals, so it should only be regarded as a pathogen if isolated as a monoculture.
- Mycobacterial infections are more common in aquatic and semi-aquatic chelonians. This is a sporadic condition that affects many different areas of the body. Palpebral oedema and exophthalmus can be seen.
- Bacterial opportunistic pathogens are usually secondary to primary ocular disease or a generalised immunosuppression. *Pseudomonas* spp., *Aeromonas* spp., *Micrococcus* spp., *Aerococcus* spp., *Staphylococcus* spp., *Corynebacterium* spp. and many of the Enterobacteriaceae have been isolated (see Figure 24.2).
- Trauma can be due to injury or it can be self-inflicted due to other ocular or periocular pathology.
- Hypovitaminosis A is most commonly seen in young, rapidly growing aquatic species fed diets deficient in vitamin A. The symptoms seen are orbital and palpebral oedema, secondary conjunctivitis and blepharitis. Treatment is oral vitamin A. The response is usually rapid, but full histological cure may take over 6 months. On occasion, antimicrobials may be required for secondary infections.
- Corneal conditions and other pathology of the eyeball can lead to conjunctivitis, oedema and blepharitis.
- UV light photokeratitis presents clinically as closed eyes, mild chemosis, blepharitis and inflammation of the skin around the eyes. More severe cases may present with skin lesions over the head and back. Signs usually appear within 1–3 days of the introduction of a new light. In man, this is a very painful condition. Symptoms usually resolve within 12–48 hours of removal of the radiation source. Bulbs causing photokeratitis have been found to be emitting UVB radiation with wavelengths below 300 nm and some have been found to be emitting UVC radiation. For further information on the safe use of UV-emitting lamps, see Chapter 2.1.

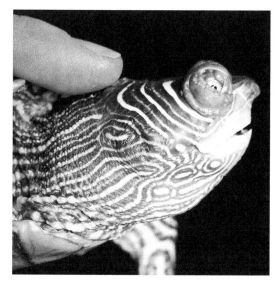

Figure 24.2    Chemosis with miliary abscessation.

- Neoplasms, although rare, can occur and be a cause of periocular, palpebral or ocular swelling.
- Orbital abscesses or any retrobulbar mass will cause exophthalmus. Depending on the size of the patient, ultrasound can be a useful diagnostic tool. If a mass is identified, an ultrasound-guided fine needle aspirate can be diagnostic. Samples are collected for cytology and culture.

## Congenital ocular malformations

Microphthalmos (small eye) occurs with some frequency in captive-bred reptiles, possibly as consequence of inbreeding or environmental conditions. Other congenital abnormalities include cyclopia (failure of the orbital fossa to divide – it may have a single central orbit and it will also have other facial abnormalities) and anophthalmos (complete absence of ocular tissue). These frequently occur with skeletal abnormalities.

# 25 Ocular Opacities and Blindness

Eye changes are common in captive Chelonia.

Ocular examination is exceptionally difficult, due to problems in restraint of the animal and the very small eye. In aquatic species, examination is further hampered by the translucent third eyelid.

In addition, the striated muscle of the reptile iris makes mydriasis much more difficult. While neuromuscular junction blocking agents may be used in the avian eye, the very small chelonian eye is not readily amenable to intracameral injection.

Therefore sedation/anaesthesia is frequently necessary for a full ocular examination, especially in aquatic species – even then, it may be difficult to achieve mydriasis and the small papillary aperture will still limit examination of the posterior segment.

However, examination of the anterior segment is possible even in the conscious animal, provided that the head can be restrained. Slit lamps suitable for mammalian species are appropriate in chelonia, though a limited examination may be performed with a conventional direct ophthalmoscope and a bright pen torch.

Fluorescein may be used to stain corneal ulcers, as in mammals.

Peri-ocular tissue examination is described elsewhere (see Chapter 24).

## Assessment of blindness

Pupillary light reflexes are often sluggish or absent even in normal animals, so these are unreliable. Similarly, corneal or threat blink reflexes are very variable between individuals.

Therefore, assessment of blindness is based on:

- observation of movement and apparent blindness – especially by the owner
- ability to find food (see below)
- finding of lesions likely to cause blindness

This latter finding includes lesions that produce obvious opacities within the eye.

Opacities may occur due to the following.

*Essentials of Tortoise Medicine and Surgery*, First Edition. John Chitty and Aidan Raftery.
© 2013 John Chitty and Aidan Raftery. Published 2013 by John Wiley & Sons, Ltd.

# Corneal changes

## Keratitis

See Figure 25.1.

### *Causes*

- Irritation or trauma.
- Cold damage (see below).
- Excessive exposure to ultraviolet light (especially to ultraviolet in the harmful UV-C range from faulty/incorrect light sources (see http://www.uvguide.co.uk):
  - infection (including chelonid herpesvirus)
  - idiopathic

### *Diagnosis*

- Examination – thick caseous crusts often form.
- Negative fluorescin staining.

### *Investigation*

- Environmental evaluation (especially ultraviolet light).
- Dietary evaluation.
- Chelonid herpesvirus PCR.
- Corneal cytology.
- Corneal bacteriology.

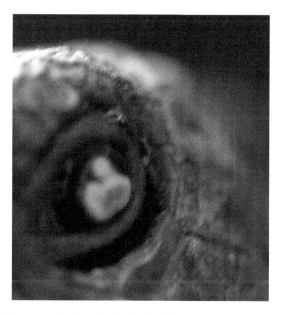

Figure 25.1    Keratitis secondary to irritation by bedding.

## *Therapy*

- Correction of environmental/dietary factors.
- Topical antibiosis.
- Topical antivirals (if indicated).
- Topical anti-inflammatories – generally non-steroidal anti-inflammatories are appropriate, though topical corticosteroids may be indicated in severe cases where there is no evidence of infection or when topical non-steroidals have been ineffective.
- Some authors advocate topical papain (papaya or pineapple juice).
- Systemic non-steroidal anti-inflammatory drugs in severe cases.
- In very severe non-responsive unilateral cases, enucleation may be considered.

## Ulceration

### *Causes*

- Irritation.
- Trauma.
- Infection.

### *Diagnosis*

- Examination.
- Positive fluorescin staining.

### *Investigation*

- Environmental evaluation (especially substrate).
- Corneal cytology and bacteriology.

### *Therapy*

- Correction of environmental factors – in particular, remove possible penetrants such as hay or straw.
- Debridement (chemical or physical) and grid keratotomy, as in mammals – anaesthesia will be required and magnification is very useful!
- Topical antimicrobial.
- Topical ketorolac (non-steroidal anti-inflammatory) in very painful cases.

## Cholesterol or lipid deposits

Cholesterol deposits are found especially in semi-aquatic species, and may be associated with high fat diets and hypercholesterolaemia/hyperlipaemia. A link to hypothyroidism may be speculated but is unproven. It may also be reported as an aging process (arcus lipoides cornea in *Testudo* species).

## Therapy

Any therapy will depend on dietary correction.

# Anterior chamber changes

These are rarely diagnosed.

## Hypopyon

Pus in the anterior chamber is often secondary to corneal ulceration/penetration. If bilateral, consider septicaemic spread, which indicates systemic investigation (haematology/biochemistry; imaging for septic foci; and 8 MHz Doppler auscultation of the heart to assess endocarditic murmurs).

## Therapy

- If ulceration of the cornea, treat as above.
- Systemic and topical antibiosis – ofloxacin is particularly useful.
- Topical non-steroidal anti-inflammatory if no ulceration.
- Enucleation if severe and non-responsive (and unilateral).

## Hyphaema

Blood in the anterior chamber is generally seen as a sequel to trauma.

If bilateral, consider a coagulopathy (haematology/biochemistry to investigate liver disorders; imaging of the liver; and investigation of possible coumarol exposure).

## Therapy

- Topical and systemic non-steroidal anti-inflammatory drugs.
- Topical corticosteroid if non-responsive and no evidence of infection.
- Topical antimicrobials.
- Therapy of any identified underlying disorders.

# Lens changes

### Cataract

See Figure 25.2. Diagnosis is based on ocular examination:

### Causes

- Cold-related: check history (see below).
- Age-related/idiopathic.
- Inflammatory – other inflammatory changes may be seen on examination.

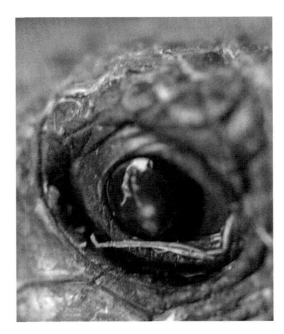

Figure 25.2    An early cataract in an elderly tortoise.

## Therapy

- Cataract removal surgery (e.g. phacoemulsification) inappropriate in small eyes.
- If no inflammation/pain, then leave alone and hand feed if necessary (see Chapter 10).
- If inflammatory changes, then consider topical and systemic anti-inflammatory drugs and antibiosis.
- If unilateral and painful, consider enucleation.
- If the tortoise is unable to feed or the inflammation is uncontrollable and bilateral, consider euthanasia.

## Cold-induced blindness

It is commonly proposed that some cases of anorexia in hibernated Mediterranean tortoises are caused by blindness. These animals are unable to find food, yet will feed if food is given directly to the mouth by hand.

The main clinical sign is a generalised opacity of the lens, similar to a cataract. The cause is due to ice crystal formation within the lens (when the hibernation temperature falls below freezing point), resulting in cellular disruption.

However, this may be difficult to comprehend, as some animals with full cataracts are able to find food and feed. This may relate to the speed of onset of the blindness.

In addition, in many groups only one or two may be affected, even though all have been exposed to low temperatures. This may also relate to individual effects, where weaker animals may not fully retract the head into the shell while hibernating. In addition, many studies show reptiles, including chelonia, often to be well adapted to cold (Muir *et al.* 2010).

Tortoises also have a very well-developed sense of smell that may be more directly useful in locating food, especially as it is very unlikely that tortoises can actually visualise the food that they are prehending, which makes it debatable how much influence blindness would have on this process (Bels *et al.* 2008).

It is also true that many apparently blind animals do not have obvious changes within the lens.

In summary, it is more probable that these cold-related cases relate to more than just blindness. The eyes and fore-brain (with olfactory lobes) are in very close apposition. Therefore, these cases may relate to a more general damage to the central nervous system than simply causing blindness. In other words, they should therefore be more fully evaluated, as there may also be more general clinical effects. It is also possible that signs may not be related to cold, but may be distinct and potentially treatable ocular problems – a full ophthalmic examination is always indicated in these cases, alongside a general clinical examination and a full husbandry review (Chapters 2.1 and 4.2).

## References

Bels, V., Baussart, S., Davenport, J., *et al.* (2008) Functional evolution of feeding behaviour in turtles. In: *Biology of Turtles* (eds J. Wyneken, M.H. Godfrey & V. Bels). CRC Press, Boca Raton, FL.

Muir T.J., Costanzo, J.P. & Lee, R.E. (2010) Brief chilling to subzero temperature increases cold hardiness in the hatchling Painted turtle (*Chrysemys picta*). *Physiological and Biochemal Zoology*, 83(1), 174–181.

# 26 Generalised Oedema or Anasarca

This is an occasionally seen sign that indicates severe disease and, generally, a guarded to poor prognosis.

However, initially this must be distinguished from body fat/obesity – especially in Horsfield's tortoises, where obese individuals will have fat deposits extending laterally from both axillae and pre-femoral fossae.

For the investigation of coelomic cavity distension, see Chapter 12.2 (see also Figure 26.1).

To some extent, the investigation is similar to that described in Chapter 37 for swelling of the fore/hind quarters, though in generalised oedema the likely diagnoses are more systemic than localised.

These can be summarised as follows:

- Circulatory failure:
  - cardiac failure
  - central lymphatic or venous occlusion
- Renal failure – especially in animals receiving systemic fluid therapy (the onset of oedema or anasarca during fluid therapy carries a poor prognosis).
- Hypoproteinaemia/hypoalbuminaemia. The causes of this are essentially the same as in other species (see Chapter 9.1):
  - intake problems –
    - malnutrition/starvation/anorexia
    - malabsorption
    - endoparasitism
  - failure to process –
    - hepatic disease
  - excess loss –
    - protein-losing nephropathy
    - protein-losing enteropathy
    - extensive skin damage
    - parasitism

*Essentials of Tortoise Medicine and Surgery*, First Edition. John Chitty and Aidan Raftery.
© 2013 John Chitty and Aidan Raftery. Published 2013 by John Wiley & Sons, Ltd.

(a)    (b)

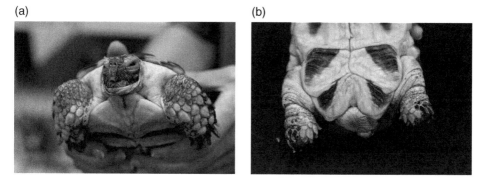

Figure 26.1    Fluid swelling of (a) forequarters and (b) hindquarters in this Hermann's tortoise.

The investigation should therefore reflect the systemic nature of these differentials:

- Clinical examination should assess, in particular:
  - body condition
  - the extent of the oedema
  - demeanour/weakness
  - the colour of the mucous membrane – pallor/cyanosis

**NB** Icterus is extremely rare, though it is easy to confuse icterus with pallor in some 'sandy-coloured' individuals, especially Horsfield's tortoises.

  - Cardiac auscultation, using an 8 MHz Doppler, may reveal heart murmurs, especially if associated with endocarditis.

- Haematology/biochemistry:
  - It should be noted that many of these cases will have extremely low red/white cell counts, as well as low protein levels. For this reason, it can be hard to differentiate between lymphodilution and a 'true' sample. In lymphodilution, there is often a proteinaceous background staining of fresh blood samples that is not seen on blood smears, and this may be the only indication. However, this staining is not always present, so the clinician may need to rely on 'instinct' in distinguishing from lymphodilution in these cases.
- Cytology and fluid analysis of any abdominal fluid – in spite of extensive oedema, this can be hard to obtain, with fluid seemingly present as extracellular fluid, making aspiration difficult.
- Faecal sample – parasitology (including fresh smear to assess faecal fauna).
- Urine sample – cytology, looking for protein 'casts' or *Spironucleus* (see Chapter 29).
- Radiography – general body views, looking for masses or foreign bodies (see Figure 26.2).
- Ultrasonography:
  - abdomen, assessing the liver, reproductive tract and possible neoplasia
  - heart
- Once oedema has reduced, coeloscopy may be attempted with care. This may enable more direct visualisation of the liver and biopsy.

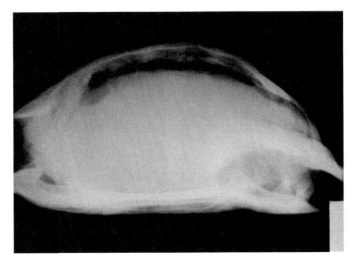

Figure 26.2   A lateral radiograph showing ascites in a tortoise with egg-related peritonitis. Ultrasonography confirmed reproductive activity. Cytology of abdominal fluid showed an inflammatory reaction – grossly egg material was visible.

## Therapy

Naturally, this should be based on treating the underlying cause.

However, some generalised principles apply:

- Biological support – heat/ultraviolet light/bathing.
- Nutrition – critical nutrition is vitally important. Good-quality protein critical feeds should be given to carnivorous species. However, these should also be used (sparingly) with higher-fibre herbivorous formulae in hypo-albuminaemic herbivorous species (see Chapter 5.4.1).
- Fluid therapy – of great importance. However, care is required when giving systemic fluids to oedematous animals – too rapid a rate of fluid dosing will worsen the situation. The intracoelomic route should be avoided in these cases.
- Phosphate binders – in renal failure where there is hyperphosphataemia.
- If faecal samples cannot be obtained, then prophylactic deworming may be indicated (see Chapter 29).
- Cardiac disease – rarely diagnosed and treated. We have used ACE inhibitors and pimobendan with little effect.
- Diuresis – if renal function is adequate, then furosemide may be used with care.

It is always important to remember the poor prognosis associated with this clinical sign and owners should be warned accordingly.

Monitoring through therapy is vital – in particular, bloods should be assessed every 5 days during therapy. If parameters worsen and clinical signs are non-progressive or worsening, then euthanasia should be considered.

# 27 Inflammation of the Oral (Stomatitis) and Pharyngeal Areas

Signs seen with stomatitis and/or pharyngeal inflammation (pharyngitis) include the following:

- Petechial haemorrhages in the mucosa.
- Ulceration.
- Necrotic exudate deposited on the tongue.
- Decrease in food intake, even if the patient is hungry.
- Difficulty swallowing (dysphagia).
- Drooling.
- Swelling.

Discharges may be seen on the oral cavity that are associated with the following:

- Upper respiratory tract infections where discharges drain into the oropharyngeal area through the choana.
- Otitis media may result in pustular material seen in the oropharyngeal area, which has come from the auditory canal.
- Lower respiratory infections may result in frothy material exiting from the glottis. This is usually accompanied by respiratory wheezy sounds and an increased respiratory rate. In some dyspnoeic cases, the glottis may be permanently open, with a frothy material visible down the trachea.
- Oesophagitis and gastritis can result in reflux of material into the oral cavity.
- Iatrogenic causes – oral enrofloxacin has been associated with regurgitation in box turtles and with hypersalivation in many species.

Investigation of stomatitis must include a full examination, a review of the husbandry, diet and past medical history, and information about all other chelonians with which it was in contact.

A haematology and biochemistry screen will help to identify underlying disease conditions. Severe systemic disease can often present as stomatitis, as a consequence of immunosuppression or secondary to hyperuricaemia.

Depending on the preliminary findings, ultrasound, endoscopy and other advanced imaging techniques may be indicated.

## Aetiology

- Viral stomatitis:
  - Herpesvirus infections are a common cause of stomatitis in a wide range of species. All species should be considered susceptible. Rhinitis, conjunctivitis, stomatitis and glossitis are common signs seen. Pathogenicity depends on the strain. Diagnosis is by PCR electron microscopy and virus isolation. Serology tests may be offered, but are not regarded as reliable. Many individuals carry a strain of herpesvirus that may not be pathogenic to them. A positive result does not confirm that it is the pathogen.
  - Ranavirus infections can cause ulcerative pharyngitis and oesophagitis in addition to rhinitis and palpebral oedema in box turtles, gopher tortoises and Burmese star tortoises, and most likely also in other species. PCR, electron microscopy and virus isolation are available. Histology may reveal intracytoplasmic inclusions in erythrocytes.
- Bacterial stomatitis is usually secondary to immunosuppression. Infections are often mixed. Common isolates include *Pseudomonas* spp., *Klebsiella* spp., *Acinetobacter* spp., *Enterobacter* spp. and *Pasteurella* spp. Treatment must include identifying the underlying cause in addition to anti-bacterial treatment, ideally based on sensitivity testing (see Figure 27.1).
- Abscesses can occur in or adjacent to the oral and pharyngeal areas, and result in stomatitis. A fine needle aspirate of any swelling is usually a rapid diagnostic test to identify the cause and obtain material for culture and sensitivity testing.
- Neoplasia is a rare but possible cause of stomatitis. Again, a fine needle aspirate is often diagnostic.

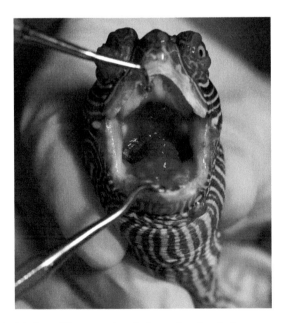

Figure 27.1    Bacterial stomatitis secondary to hypovitaminosis A.

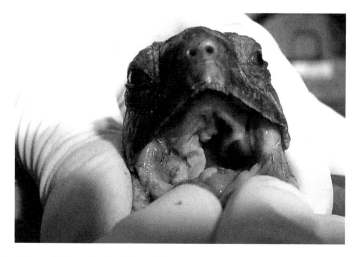

Figure 27.2    Stomatitis and glossitis, with caesous necrotic plaques building up in the oral cavity.

- Hypovitaminosis A is a possible cause of stomatitis. It leads to abnormal keratinisation of the mucosa (and other areas of the body), which can predispose to stomatitis and respiratory infections.
- Chemical irritants can be the cause of acute onset stomatitis.
- Trauma from a predator or local irritation from rough food.
- Map turtles (*Graptemys* spp.) are highly adapted to a diet containing a high proportion of snails with hard shells. If these are excluded from the diet, the oral mucosa can become thickened (see Figure 27.2).

## Treatment

- Optimal environmental conditions are essential for recovery.
- Fluid replacement therapy by the oral, intra-osseous route as a continuous infusion or epicoelomic boluses.
- Anti-bacterials for the opportunist secondary bacterial infections.
- Nutritional support either by stomach tubing if short term or via an oesophageal feeding tube if needed in the longer term.
- The cleaning of necrotic debris from the oral and nasal cavity with cotton tips as required.
- Quarantine from other chelonians may need to be lifelong depending on the pathogen identified.
- Antivirals have been used with variable reported results for herpesvirus infections. Acyclovir at 80 mg/kg three times daily by oral gavage has been reported to have a positive effect if started early in the disease course. A dose rate of 80 mg/kg q72 hours is also proposed (see Appendix 1). Acyclovir should only be used in confirmed cases, due to the risk of side effects. If the individual recovers from a herpesvirus infection it, and all other in-contact individuals, should be regarded as infected for life and permanently quarantined.

# 28 External Parasites

In the United Kingdom, other than in newly imported (or those in contact), ectoparasites (barring myiasis) are extremely unusual.

Species that may be encountered include the following.

## Flies

### Calliphorid and sarcophagid flies

Many species are linked to myiasis (see Figure 28.1). Primary causes are usually wounds or prolapses (entry via *Amblyomma* spp. tick wounds has been recorded in gopher tortoises) and debility. The prognosis for myiasis is poor – partly due to the need to address the underlying cause (which is often severe) as well as difficulties removing maggots and treating those left behind (avermectins are contraindicated in Chelonia). Physical removal and flushing (0.05% chlorhexidine recommended) are essential to remove maggots. F10 preparations, including cypermethrin and piperonyl butoxide (Health & Hygiene Pty, SA), permethrin 0.01% and fipronil, have also been used to repel maggots from wounds. Fluid and thermal support are essential due to the probable toxic state post-myiasis (and to assist in supporting probable underlying debility).

Prevention involves avoidance of underlying causes and detection of these cases before they strike (another reason for poor prognosis is that the strike is often not detected for a long time), good husbandry (prevention of the build-up of organic material and maintenance of adequate environmental temperature – see Chapter 2.1) and regular checking of pet chelonians.

### Biting flies

*Aedes* and *Glossina* spp. have been recorded as feeding on turtles and leopard tortoises, respectively. Clinically, they have little effect on reptiles other than heavy loads causing blood loss and debility in very small animals. In Africa, *Glossina* spp.

*Essentials of Tortoise Medicine and Surgery*, First Edition. John Chitty and Aidan Raftery.
© 2013 John Chitty and Aidan Raftery. Published 2013 by John Wiley & Sons, Ltd.

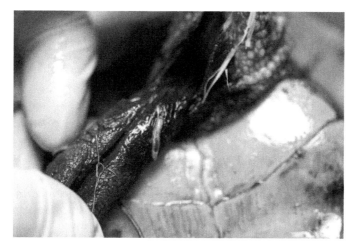

Figure 28.1    Myiasis of a prolapsed hemipene.

are implicated in the spread of trypanosomiasis. Control is via treatment/reduction of standing water for fly breeding in areas close to the reptiles. If a problem, dichlorvos-impregnated strips may be suspended in the reptile room though care must be taken to avoid contact with reptiles and people as toxicity can be an issue.

## Ticks

### *Haemaphysalis, Hyalomma, Amblyomma, Aponomma and Ornithodoros* spp.

A variety of hard and soft tick species have been recorded in Chelonia. These are generally found in the recesses in front of the hind or fore legs. There is often no reaction or clinical consequence, though large numbers may cause problems due to blood loss. Skin reactions may occasionally be seen. Ticks have also been implicated in the spread of haemoparasites. More importantly, some of these species can also parasitise man, and can spread relapsing fever and heartwater. It is therefore important when importing chelonians that an adequate quarantine period, with regular thorough checks, is undertaken. Permethrin and fipronil sprays appear to be effective in removing ticks and, in quarantine, should be employed prophylactically.

# 29 Internal Parasites

The following parasites may be encountered in captive Chelonia. In general, the herbivorous species appear more prone to endoparasitism than carnivorous. In herbivorous species, there is also a need to distinguish between commensal organisms and pathogenic ones (see below) – in all cases it is also important to assess relative numbers of organisms (compared with clinical signs), as some species may be *potential* pathogens and may only cause problems if allowed to overgrow the gut.

## Protozoa

### Haemoprotozoa

The following have been described in Chelonia:

- *Chelonoplasma* spp. (see Figure 29.1)
- *Haemoproteus* spp. (aka *Simondia* spp.)
- *Trypanosoma* spp.
- *Aegyptionella* spp. (aka *Tunetella* spp.)
- Coccidians – *Haemogregarina* spp., *Haemohormidium guglielmi*
- *Nuttallia* spp.
- Rickettsia – *Grahamella* and *Haemobartonella* spp.
- *Plasmodium* spp.

All are transmitted by the bite of arthropod (or leech, in aquatic species) vectors.

The vast majority of these parasites have not been associated with any clinical signs in the host animal. However, the presence of the parasite in blood smears does indicate previous exposure to the appropriate vector (generally, in temperate countries this means that the animal has been imported) and the presence of large numbers of parasites may indicate stress or debility and immunocompromise in the host.

However, the following have been associated with clinical signs:

- *Chelonoplasma* spp. – subcutaneous small haemorrhages in ventro-lateral aspects of the legs and tail of the host

*Essentials of Tortoise Medicine and Surgery*, First Edition. John Chitty and Aidan Raftery.
© 2013 John Chitty and Aidan Raftery. Published 2013 by John Wiley & Sons, Ltd.

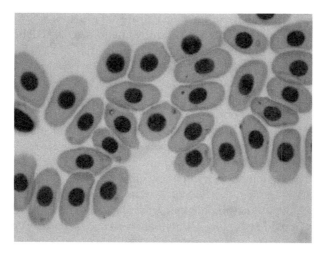

Figure 29.1    Chelonoplasma inclusions in red cells. Courtesy of Nick Carmichael, CTDS Lab Ltd.

- *Plasmodium* spp. – heavy parasite burdens may cause anaemia due to erythrocyte destruction
- *Haemogregarina* spp. – may be associated with anaemia and inappetance

Diagnosis of these parasites is by examination of fresh air-dried blood smears. Identification of these parasites is difficult, as many are poorly classified and easily confused with other cell inclusions or artefacts. Therefore, the use of anti-coagulated blood for smears is not recommended. It is advised that such smears should be submitted to a haematologist who is experienced with Chelonia.

Therapy for haemoparasitism has not been reliably described, presumably due to the rarity of clinically significant infection, though toltrazuril is reported as effective against coccidians. However, the finding of large numbers of these parasites does indicate a need for supportive care.

## Coccidia

- Intranuclear coccidians have been associated with disease in *Geochelone radiata*, *G. pardalis*, *Indotestudo forsteni* and *Manouria impressa*:
  - ○ Signs included profound weakness and debility – clinical pathology indicated anaemia and renal compromise.
  - ○ Post-mortem examination indicated nephritis, enteritis, pancreatitis and hepatitis.
  - ○ Oocysts did not appear to be shed in faeces. Therefore, this would appear to be a post-mortem diagnosis, or one based on histopathology of organ biopsies.
  - ○ Toltrazuril could be presumed to be a possible treatment, though this was not attempted in the described cases.
- *Eimeria* spp. have been described in the gastrointestinal tract of many species (terrestrial and semi-aquatic). Presumably these species are specific to the host

species/genus and site as in other animal groups. They appear not to be associated with any clinical signs, though may contribute to a general debilitation:

o   Oocysts can be readily identified in faecal floats.

o   Toltrazuril is an effective treatment.

- *Sarcocystis* spp. and *Isospora* spp. have also been described in Chelonia, though not associated with clinical signs.
- *Cryptosporidium* spp. – these have been described in many species of tortoise and semi-aquatic turtle, but are rarely associated with disease. However, there are occasional reports of association with gastritis and regurgitation. In one case (*Testudo kleinmanni*), cryptosporidiosis was associated with coelomitis and ascites, following an overwhelming enteritis:

o   Diagnosis is by identification of oocysts in faeces or (better) gastric/cloacal washes. Oocysts may be identified by phase contrast microscopy on faecal floats or by acid-fast stains. Immunofluorescence assays may be more sensitive.

o   A suggested screening for carriers is by checking three samples, 3–5 days apart.

o   Care should be taken when screening semi-aquatic species – *Mantonella hammondi* has been reported as a 'passenger'/pseudo-parasite in the faeces of yellow mud turtles. It is normally regarded as a parasite of invertebrates.

o   No effective therapies have been described. In an outbreak, positive animals should be removed from a collection.

## Flagellates

The following have been described in Chelonia:

- *Spironucleus* spp. (aka *Hexamita* spp.)
- Trichomonads
- *Giardia* spp.
- *Leptomonas* spp.
- *Trepomonas* spp.
- *Monocercomonoides* spp.
- *Proteomonas* spp.
- *Chilomastix* spp.
- *Retortamonas* spp.
- *Hypotrichomonas* spp.

With the exception of *Hypotrichomonas* (enteritis) and *Spironucleus*, none are associated with clinical signs, and small numbers should be expected as normal in fresh faecal samples/washes and urine from all Chelonia. However, in debilitated individuals, overgrowth of flagellates may be seen with an associated enteritis.

In these cases, a single dose of metronidazole may be effective. However, attention must be paid to restocking this gut fauna with subsequent feeding of fresh faeces from clinically normal animals of the same species (preferably from the same collection).

*Spironucleus* has been described as causing anorexia weight loss and renal failure, as a slowly progressive disease in a number of species. However, it is proposed that it is only potentially pathogenic in association with other pathogens. Renal biopsy is required for diagnosis of clinical spironucleosis. Therapy is as above.

It is also important to remember that some of these organisms may be pathogens in other species – for example, *Leptomonas* causing colitis in chameleons.

Therefore, attention must be paid to preventing cross-contamination in mixed reptile collections.

## Other protozoa

### Ciliates

*Balantidium* spp. and *Nyctotherus* spp. are normal findings in fresh faecal samples and cloacal washes from all Chelonia.

They do not appear to be associated with clinical disease unless there is overgrowth and enteritis in a debilitated individual. Diagnosis and management is as for flagellates (see above).

### Entamoeba spp.

A variety of *Entamoeba* spp. parasitise the gut of different chelonian species. These are not associated with clinical signs.

However, *E. invadens* may be found as a commensal in herbivorous terrestrial Chelonia – this may cause enteritis in snakes and carnivorous lizards. Care, therefore, must be taken when keeping these species in mixed collections. Herbivorous chelonians may be screened for this organism by direct smears from fresh faeces or cloacal washes. While metronidazole may be effective in treating entamoebiasis, it is not clear if it is effective in clearing the organism without damaging the gut microfauna.

Strict quarantine and biosecurity between species is, therefore, more appropriate.

### Toxoplasma spp.

Tissue cysts have been reported in various chelonians, though no clinical signs have been reported. It is unclear whether or not these *Toxoplasma* species are related to those infecting mammals.

### Sessilids

*Epistyles* and *Opercularia* spp. have been reported attached to the skin of soft-shelled turtles. However, clinical signs have not been reported.

### Acanthamoeba and Endolimax spp.

These are found in the intestine of freshwater turtles and box turtles, and are not associated with clinical signs.

However, *Acanthamoeba* may be associated with neurological disease in snakes. As described earlier, care must therefore be taken to avoid cross-contamination in mixed reptile collections.

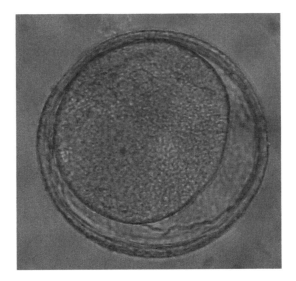

Figure 29.2   Ascarid ovum.

## Nematodes

### Ascarids

Commonly found in captive Chelonia (see Figure 29.2).

Direct and indirect life cycles – therefore once in a colony, may be difficult to eradicate.

Direct clinical signs are unusual, though they may cause the following:

- gastrointestinal obstruction (large, up to 10 cm long adults)
- vomition
- wasting
- intussusception
- gastrointestinal ulceration and peritonitis
- larval migration may be associated with pulmonary lesions
- a single case has reported larvae-associated ear abscess in *Testudo graeca*

However, more commonly they may be contributors to disease in debilitated animals or those with sub-optimal husbandry.

Diagnosis is by finding eggs in faecal floats or in stomach washings.

Therapy involves one of the following:

- benzimidazoles
- emodepsid
- levamisole – though reports on the effectiveness of this drug are varied and conflicting
- **DO NOT USE IVERMECTIN!**

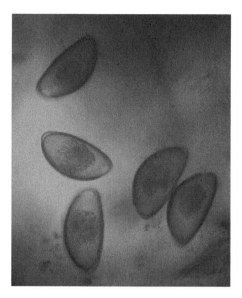

Figure 29.3    Oxyurid ova.

Prevention is by good husbandry and/or routine deworming – see later.

## Proatractis

Adult worms 0.5–1.0 cm in length found in large intestine.

Direct life cycle.

May cause anorexia and lethargy. Have been associated with fatal syndrome in *Geochelone carbonaria*.

Diagnosis by faecal flotation. However, as viviparous, Baermann flotation may be required to identify larvae. For this reason, fresh faeces must be used to avoid confusion with hatched larvae in older faecal samples.

Therapy – conventional anthelmintics appear to be ineffective.

## Oxyurids

Very common in captive herbivorous Chelonia – especially *Testudo* spp. (see Figure 29.3).

Adults found in large intestine.

Direct life cycle, so hard to eradicate from a colony.

Unlikely to directly cause disease, though severe infections have been linked to rectal prolapse and to intestinal obstruction. However, may be major contributors to disease (especially anorexia syndromes) in debilitated individuals or those kept in sub-optimal husbandry. For these reasons, pet owners in the UK are often advised to use routine deworming therapy.

Diagnosis – identification of eggs in faecal floats.

Therapy and prevention – see ascarids and later.

**DO NOT USE IVERMECTIN!**

## Spirurids

Adult worms found in body cavities and subcutaneous tissues.

Larvae exit via the skin and may cause pustular skin lesions.

Diagnosis is by identification of larvae in histopathological or cytological preparations from skin lesions.

Benzimidazoles may be effective, but as relatively non-pathogenic, occasional skin lesions may be treated symptomatically.

**DO NOT USE IVERMECTIN!**

## Cestodes

Extremely uncommon, though reported in aquatic and semi-aquatic freshwater species.

Non-pathogenic.

## Pentastomids

May be found in the lungs of some aquatic species, where an inflammatory reaction may occur.

As they require an intermediate host in their life cycle, these are only found in wild-caught individuals.

## Trematodes – spirorchiids

A variety of fluke species may infect Chelonia (see Figure 29.4). In terrestrial and aquatic species, monogeneans (direct life cycle) may inhabit the bladder and are considered non-pathogenic.

Digenean flukes (indirect life cycle) may infect aquatic species, with adult flukes being found in many organs, including the heart ventricles. Eggs, similarly, are found encysted in many organs and also in the faeces. Clinical signs, surprisingly, are unusual, though disease has been reported in freshwater turtles, with signs including lethargy, altered swimming patterns, hemiplegia and shell ulceration. Obviously, given the need for an intermediate host in the parasite life cycle,

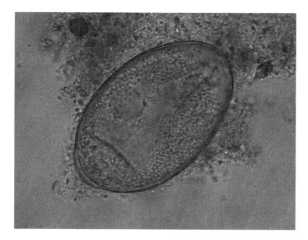

Figure 29.4    Fluke ovum.

this will only be seen in wild-caught individuals or in animals fed on wild-taken food sources.

Diagnosis is generally on post-mortem examination and histopathology of infected tissues, though faecal flotation may reveal typical eggs.

For animals fed on wild-taken prey, care must be taken to distinguish potentially pathogenic trematode eggs from those of the prey – that is, pseudo-parasites.

## Acanthocephalans

'Spiny headed worms', found commonly in wild semi-aquatic/aquatic freshwater species. Adults are found in the intestine, while encapsulated larvae are found in the intestinal wall.

While intestinal occlusion may occur, these are generally considered non-pathogenic.

As with pathogenic trematodes, these have an indirect life cycle and so, in captivity, are generally only likely to be found in wild-caught individuals.

## Prophylactic anthelmintic therapy

It is frequently debated whether or not anti-parasitic prophylaxis should be performed.

In an ideal clinical world, all deparasitising should be based on full assessment of the level of parasitism and species involved (see earlier). This will determine the need for dosing and the appropriate drug to use.

However, in some cases, as in other areas of clinical medicine, the situation (based on previous disease history, parasite levels, stocking levels and, to a lesser extent, financial means) may indicate that routine deworming may be employed.

It should be noted, however, that where benzimidazoles are used routinely:

- There is some risk of toxic side-effects (see Appendix 1), though these appear rare in clinical practice.
- Fenbendazole requires conversion to oxfendazole for its activity – therefore, if the chelonian is not at adequate temperature/health, then it may not be able to convert the drug efficiently and a single dose will be ineffective. If used as single doses, it may be more appropriate to use oxfendazole.
- Benzimidazoles act by paralysing the nematodes. Therefore, treated tortoises will pass still-moving worms for (up to) several weeks after deworming. Concerned owners should be assured that the passing of the worms is a sign of efficacy, *not* a requirement for further dosing. If in doubt, a faecal screen will reveal the presence of ova – that is, whether or not there are still breeding adults in the gut.
- Care should be taken that benzimidazoles are given at the correct dose rate in order to avoid the build-up of resistance in the parasite population. Given the lack of efficacy/potential toxicity of other anthemintic classes, there are few alternatives to benzimidazoles, though a combination of emodepside and praziquantel (Profender, Bayer UK) has been shown to be efficacious against nematodes by topical application at 2 ml/kg (Brames 2008). This makes it a useful alternative to benzimidazoles and a likely first-choice therapy in animals where oral dosing of drugs by stomach tube is extremely difficult; for example, giant tortoises. It should also be noted that benzimidazoles may also not be without side-effects, so excessive use and over-dosing should be avoided (Neiffer *et al.* 2005). However, it is not clear whether these effects are seen with all benzimidazoles or only fenbendazole, which acts as a pro-drug.

## References

Brames, H. (2008) Efficacy and tolerability of profender in reptiles: spot-on treatment against nematodes. *Exotic DVM*, **10**(3), 29–34.
Neiffer, D.L., Lydick, D., Burks, K. & and Doherty, D. (2005) Hematologic and plasma biochemical changes associated with fenbendazole administration in Hermann's tortoises (*Testudo hermanni*). *Journal of Zoo and Wildlife Medicine*, **36**(4), 661–672.

## Further reading

Barnard, S.M. & Upton, S.J. (1994) *A Veterinary Guide to the Parasites of Reptiles*, vol. 1, *Protozoa*. Krieger, Malabar, FL.
Frye, F.L. (1991) *Biomedical and Surgical Aspects of Captive Reptile Husbandry*. Krieger, Malabar, FL.
Greiner, E.C. & Mader, D.R. (2006) Parasitology. In: *Reptile Medicine and Surgery* (ed. D.R. Mader), 2nd edn, pp. 343–364. Saunders, St Louis, MO.
Jacobsen, E.R. (2007) Parasites and parasitic diseases of reptiles. In: *Infectious Diseases and Pathology of Reptiles* (ed. E.R. Jacobsen), pp. 571–666. Taylor & Francis, Boca Raton, FL.
McArthur, S., Wilkinson, R. & Meyer, J. (2004) *Medicine and Surgery of Tortoises and Turtles*. Blackwell, Oxford.

# 30  Peeling Skin or Shell

This is a common reason for presentation of captive chelonians. As with many of the other problems described in this book, the major problem can be in distinguishing the pathological condition from normal physiological changes.

While the shell is, essentially, a specialised skin adnexa, such that there are many causes in common for peeling skin or shells, it is simpler to regard these as separate areas for the purposes of investigation.

## Skin

### Terrestrial species

The most likely diagnosis is of normal skin shedding, especially in young animals. However, this should be external skin layers only and there should be no sign of inflammation/ulceration (see Figure 30.1). Should there be inflammation or ulceration (see Chapter 33), then the principal differentials are as follows:

a. trauma (indicated in history?)
b. infection – bacterial/fungal
c. vitamin A deficiency – check the dietary/supplement history (note that this is quite an unusual differential)
d. vitamin A toxicosis – especially if there is history of recent overdosage, particularly post-injection
e. a very localised reaction may be seen following ectoparasite attachment – there should be a history of recent import

### *Investigation*

- History (see Chapters 2.1 and 4.2).
- Examination – both systemic and dermatological (including a thorough parasite check).
- Environmental assessment (see Chapter 2.1) – in particular, hygiene, overuse of disinfectants (or other potential irritants) and nutrition should be evaluated.

*Essentials of Tortoise Medicine and Surgery*, First Edition. John Chitty and Aidan Raftery.
© 2013 John Chitty and Aidan Raftery. Published 2013 by John Wiley & Sons, Ltd.

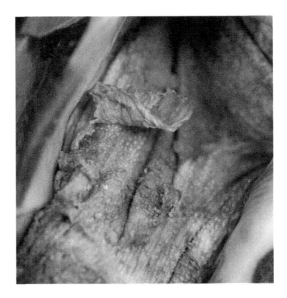

Figure 30.1    Normal skin shed in a juvenile Hermann's tortoise.

## Sampling

- Skin scrape and impression smear. These are performed as in dogs or cats. Stain for infectious disease investigation (see Chapter 5.7). A cytological response should be seen to infectious elements. Bacteria or yeast seen without a cytological response are unlikely to be significant unless found in monoculture.
- Swab for bacteriology – results should always be interpreted in association with cytology.
- Bloods – a haematology and biochemistry screen, together with an assessment of underlying disease, especially if there are generalised skin lesions.
- Biopsy – excisional or punch.

## Therapy

Always correct underlying causes where identified.

If infection (bacterial or fungal) is identified – then use an appropriate systemic anti-microbial (based on culture) alongside topical povidone-iodine or F10SC (1:250 dilution) or chlorhexidine. Silver sulphadiazine cream may be applied after daily bathing.

If Vitamin A deficiency is diagnosed on biopsy, then give long-term oral vitamin A supplement and correct diet.

Vitamin A toxicity cases are treated symptomatically alongside management of secondary infections.

## Aquatic species

These are much more likely to be related to infection secondary to poor water quality (see Chapter 2.1). Shedding problems are very unlikely, so a disease process is more likely than interpretation as a normal finding.

The principal differential diagnoses are as follows:

a. bacterial/fungal disease secondary to water-quality issues (in general, bacterial infections appear more common)
b. trauma (should be indicated in history)
c. vitamin A deficiency – as in terrestrial species, these are quite unusual
d. deficiency of essential amino acids or a poor-quality protein diet
e. vitamin A toxicosis – should be a history of recent overdosage

Ectoparasites are extremely unlikely.

### Investigation

- History (see Chapters 2.1 and 4.2).
- Examination – both systemic and dermatological.
- Environmental assessment, including water quality.
- Feeding – is the animal fed in its normal tank, or removed to a separate feeding area (i.e. is there a likelihood of increased environmental contamination?). Diet evaluation is important to check complete foods or frozen food items for expiry date and spoilage.

### Sampling

- Blood sampling – haematology/biochemistry (assessment of underlying disease).
- Lesion biopsy – excision or punch biopsy appropriate both for histopathology and culture/sensitivity. Superficial impression smears and bacteriological swabbing are inappropriate, as there is such a high likelihood of external contamination.

### Therapy

Always correct underlying causes where identified.

Dry docking of semi-aquatic species (see Chapter 3.3.1) should be utilised in all cases, as it is easier to control the environment and prevent further contamination of lesions. Fully aquatic species require pristine water quality and daily water changes.

Where infection is identified, appropriate systemic anti-microbials based on culture/sensitivity should be given.

Topical cleaning (e.g. povidone iodine or F10SC, 1:250 dilution, or chlorhexidine) should be instigated on a daily basis – apply with a soft toothbrush, followed by barrier cream (e.g. silver suphadiazine cream).

Vitamin A deficiency or excess are managed as in terrestrial species.

Diet should be corrected as per findings on evaluation, paying particular attention to protein quality.

## Shell

### Terrestrial species

This is rarely seen – if seen, treat as 'shell infection' (see Chapter 32).

### Aquatic species

#### Soft-shelled species

Treat as 'skin peeling' (see above).

#### Other aquatic species

Almost all cases relate to dysecdysis (see Figures 30.2 and 30.3) and are secondary to inappropriate environment or poor water quality. Therefore, thorough environmental assessment and correction are required (see Chapter 2.1). See also Chapter 35. Peeling layers can be removed by daily cleaning with a soft brush and chlorhexidine or povidone-iodine or F10SC (1:250 dilution) to prevent secondary infection.

In non-responsive cases (4 weeks or more) or where there are obvious inflammatory changes associated with lesions, treat as per 'skin peeling' (see above). Deep

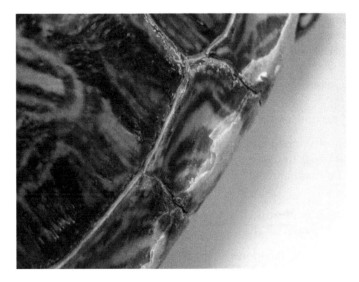

Figure 30.2    Dysecdysis in a Red-eared slider: note the edges of retained scutes.

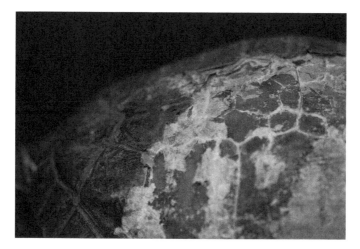

Figure 30.3   Dysecdsis in a Red-eared slider: note the multiple layers of scute and the crumbling edges of infected keratin layers.

biopsies should be taken for culture/sensitivity and histopathology, using Jamshidi bone biopsy needles. Therapy is as per 'skin peeling' – though it should be considered that healing will take longer – and if extensive, the prognosis is poor. Dry docking will always be required during the treatment period.

# 31  Prolapse

Optimal management relies on identification of the prolapsed tissue and a clinical assessment of the underlying cause, in addition to an evaluation of the viability of the tissue. This will allow a treatment plan to be formulated and a realistic prognosis to be given:

- Attempt to identify the tissue prolapsing through the vent opening (see Table 31.1).
- Collect a full history.
- Evaluate the environment and diet for the species.
- Do a full clinical examination (see Figure 31.1).
- Collect samples for haematology, biochemistry screen and faecal parasitology.

Conditions that can predispose to prolapse (see Figure 31.2):

- dystocia
- hypocalcaemia
- intestinal parasites
- uroliths
- cloacaliths
- neoplasia
- neurological deficit
- a space-occupying lesion in the coelomic cavity, causing straining

A prolapsed copulatory organ can also be caused by:

- mating injury (see Figure 31.3)
- foreign body damage (e.g. substrate sticking to an engorged organ)

Immediate treatment (depending on the needs of the patient):

- analgesia
- thermal support
- gentle flushing of the prolapsed tissue with saline (warmed to between 28 and 32 °C)
- wrapping in a moist dressing to prevent desiccation – owners can be told to protect it during transit with cling film

*Essentials of Tortoise Medicine and Surgery*, First Edition. John Chitty and Aidan Raftery.
© 2013 John Chitty and Aidan Raftery. Published 2013 by John Wiley & Sons, Ltd.

**Table 31.1** The key to identifying the prolapsed tissue

| Structure | Identification | Actions |
|---|---|---|
| Cloacal tissue | Solid tissue, no lumen <br><br> Large structure <br><br> Urates often seen coming from ureter openings | Identify that ureters are viable. They enter the urodeum of the cloaca at approximately the 10 and 2 o'clock positions. <br><br> Replace and keep in the cloaca by narrowing the vent with suture transverse mattress or simple interrupted sutures on each side of the vent. The suture must go deep, to the sphincter muscle ring. The vent is more of a slit, so purse-string sutures are less suitable. |
| Colon <br> Intestinal intussusception | Lumen present <br><br> Smooth surface <br><br> Faecal material and gas may be present in lumen | Replace if viable and keep in place by narrowing the vent as above, under cloacal tissue prolapse. This may make it difficult to monitor whether the prolapse has reoccurred internally. If there is any doubt, radiography and/or ultrasound may be indicated. <br><br> A coeliotomy is often necessary to reduce and evaluate what is viable and facilitate colopexy. With an intussusception, a coeliotomy is essential. <br><br> Amputation of an exposed devitalised section can be achieved by placing a smooth tubular object in the lumen and transfixing with hypodermic needles to keep it in place while the devitalised area is removed and the incisions anastomosed. Take care that the cloacal tissues are not incorporated in the sutures. |
| Copulatory organ | Solid mass, no lumen <br><br> Median groove may be visible <br><br> More fleshy distally | Replace and keep in the cloaca by narrowing the vent as described above, under cloacal tissue prolapse. <br><br> Amputate if devitalised or if reoccurring. <br><br> Mattress sutures placed at the base. |
| Oviduct | Longitudinal striations seen if not too devitalised <br><br> Lumen present <br><br> No faecal material | Amputate devitalised sections initially. <br><br> A coeliotomy is required to remove the remaining oviduct and ovary. <br><br> The normal side may be left; however, removal of both sides recommended. |
| Bladder | Thin translucent wall <br><br> May contain coelomic fluid | Fluid has to be removed first, by milking back into the coelomic cavity. <br><br> If viable, can be reduced manually. <br><br> An incision extending the vent opening laterally often improves visibility for full reduction. <br><br> Small non-viable sections can be removed and an inverting suture pattern used for closure. However, a seal is difficult to obtain and most cases require a coeliotomy for either partial or complete resection of the bladder. Sutures outside the lumen (placed from a coeliotomy) provide a better seal and heal with fewer complications. |

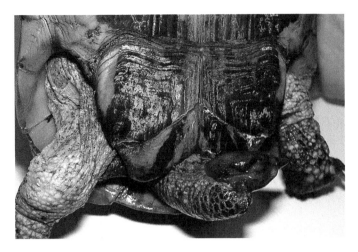

Figure 31.1   An engorged phallus, extending through the vent. This is normal and it should retract on its own.

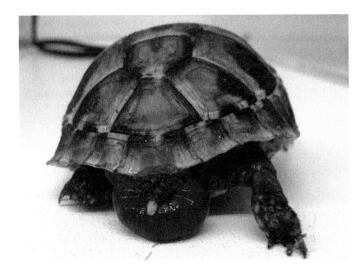

Figure 31.2   Oedematous cloacal prolapse.

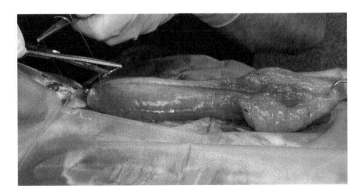

Figure 31.3   Amputation of a prolapsed phallus of this size requires careful surgery.

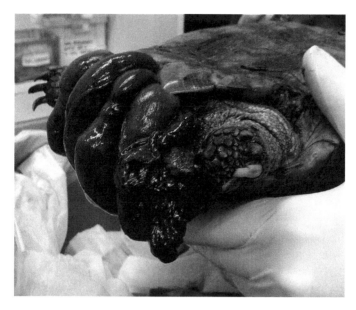

Figure 31.4   Prolapse of the colon.

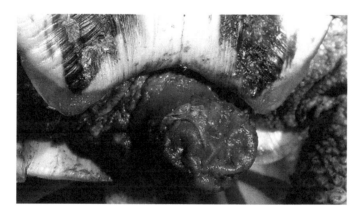

Figure 31.5   Prolapse of an intestinal intussception.

- anti-bacterial drugs
- fluids
- nutritional support
- refer promptly if a definitive diagnosis cannot be made, or if the necessary intervention is not available (see Figure 31.4)

Identification of the tissue prolapsing through the vent opening can be difficult depending on its condition, but is essential to treatment planning. Many cases are seen where the prolapse is placed back into the cloaca and a purse-string suture applied, leaving the animal with a prolonged painful death (see Figures 31.5 and 31.6).

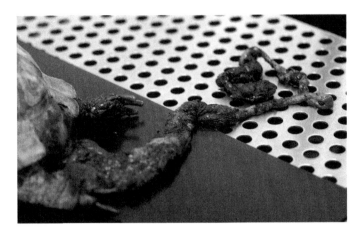

Figure 31.6   Oviduct prolapse. After stabilisation and amputation of the prolapse using a reefing technique, a coeliotomy removed the stump internally.

The haematology, biochemistry screen and faecal parasitology are to identify underlying causes of the prolapse. Radiography, ultrasound and/or cloacoscopy are often needed to identify the tissue and help with the prognosis.

**NB** Post-surgical monitoring is very important.

Hospitalise any chelonian after treatment of a prolapse for close monitoring to ensure that the returned tissue remains viable and that the prolapse does not reoccur, hidden inside the animal.

# 32 Shell Disease

## Anatomy

- The shell is living, metabolically active tissue.
- The shell is generally divided into three areas:
  - the carapace, the dorsal section of the shell
  - the plastron, the ventral section
  - the bridge across the lateral areas, which joins the carapace to the plastron
- The shell is bone covered with a thin layer of keratinised epithelium.
- The bone is made up of bony plates called dermal plates, joined together at the sutures.
- The shell bone is fused to the ribs and the vertebral bodies. In some species, it is fused to the limb girdles.
- Some of the bony plates can be used as a site to collect bone marrow – for example, the plates underlying the gular scutes, where there is a large bone marrow cavity bilaterally. They can also be used to administer intra-osseous fluids.
- Keratinised epidermal scutes cover the bony dermal plates. The areas where the scutes join are called seams.
- Growth occurs from the seam.
- The seams of the epidermal scutes do not line up with the sutures of the bony plates.
- The number and size of scutes vary with the species and are used to identify species.
- Aquatic and semi-aquatic hard-shelled species regularly shed scutes throughout life (see Figure 30.3).

## Disease presentations

- Rough, pitted keratin layers, with areas of keratin loss. Most commonly limited to the superficial layers, but sometimes also involving the underlying bone. This is a common clinical presentation in aquatic and semi-aquatic chelonians. Many pathogens (bacterial and fungal) have been associated with these changes (see Figure 32.2).

*Essentials of Tortoise Medicine and Surgery*, First Edition. John Chitty and Aidan Raftery.
© 2013 John Chitty and Aidan Raftery. Published 2013 by John Wiley & Sons, Ltd.

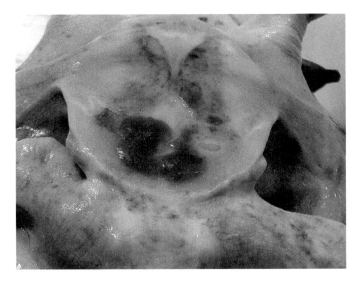

Figure 32.1   Septicaemia causing dilation and fragility of the blood vessels, resulting in hyperaemic areas.

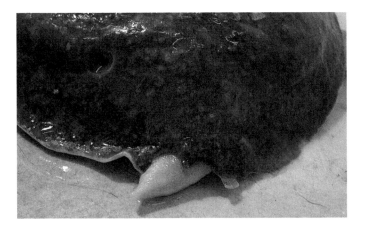

Figure 32.2   The same animal as in Figure 32.1. There were multiple deep ulcers on the carapace.

- Ulcerative shell lesions, with sloughing of scutes. The underlying bone may be just affected superficially or the lesions may invade deeper into the bone. If the lesion is deep enough, the pleuroperitoneal/coelomic membrane may be thickened, and infection may track along it. *Serratia* species have been implicated as primary pathogens in shell infection, due to their proteolytic action on tissues, allowing other potential pathogens to invade (Jackson & Fulton 1970). *Citrobacter* species are also commonly isolated from these lesions, in addition to a variety of other bacterial and fungal pathogens (see Figure 32.3).
- Retention of scutes is often seen as a presenting sign in semi-aquatic species. This is a secondary problem, often related to husbandry deficiencies; for example, tem-

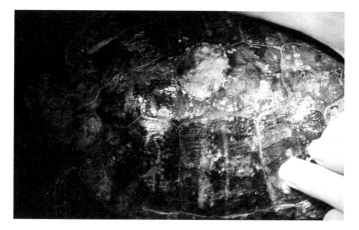

Figure 32.3    Deep debriding of this area of osteomyelitis.

perature range, basking opportunity, nutritional status and light cycle. Retained scutes are at risk of secondary infections. Retention of scutes needs to be differentiated from the normal animal that is presented as the scutes are being shed.

- Haemorrhage or red areas under scutes or along scute seams is usually indicative of sepsis, but normal coloration or focal infection must be ruled out as well. Abrasive floors and hot concrete patios are benign causes of red areas on the plastron.
- Exposed bone is sometimes seen when there is damage to the overlying scute. If localised with no evidence of an active lesion, treatment is not warranted and normal shell may regrow or a pseudoshell may form under the damaged bone.
- Soft shell can be caused by severe secondary nutritional hyperparathyroidism. Severe septicaemias can present with generalised shell softening, and a generalised reddening of the plastron with generalised oedema. There is often concurrent renal failure (see Figure 32.1).
- Localised trauma can also cause haemorrhage under the scutes. This is often caused by bite wounds that have not managed to penetrated. There are usually other areas where bite wounds are obvious.
- Neonatal turtles normally have soft shells, which gradually become firm over 6–12 months (see Figure 32.4).

## Causes of shell infection

- Most cases are probably predisposed to by husbandry factors: water quality and temperature, nutritional status, basking opportunity and other concurrent disease.
- The bacterium *Benekea chitinovora* has been shown to be a primary infectious cause of progressive superficial shell lesions, leading to mortality (Wallach 1975).
- Shell trauma can provide a route of inoculation.
- Hematogenous spread of septic thrombi appears to be the cause in some cases.

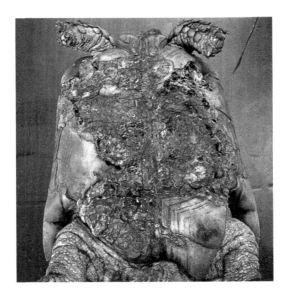

Figure 32.4   Extensive osteomyelitis destroying the plastron.

## Approach

- The environmental history should be investigated:
  - Water-quality parameters are important for aquatic and semi-aquatic chelonians. This includes temperature, pH, ammonia and nitrite content.
  - The basking zone must achieve adequate temperatures for the species. UV lighting in aquatic and semi-aquatic chelonian species that are able to absorb vitamin D from their food will have an antimicrobial effect on the carapace.
  - An inadequate diet will lead to immunosuppression and may cause nutritional metabolic bone disease.
- The history of in-contact animals, social groupings, previous illness and treatment.
- Clinical examination of all body systems, paying particular attention to the shell and skin.
- The lesions should be investigated by gently lifting loose scutes using probes. Necrotic material can be removed to assess the depth of the lesion. Sometimes it extends to the pleuroperitoneal membrane. Sometimes it is more superficial and can be found to be underrunning the scutes.
- A haematology and biochemistry screen will help to evaluate for evidence of systemic disease.
- Blood culture may be helpful, especially if the lesions are due to septic thrombi.
- Cytology, culture and histology of samples from deep in the lesion. Superficial sampling may just sample the bacteria normally found on the skin.
- Radiographs may demonstrate focal radiolucent areas secondary to abscesses. Gastrointestinal tract gas can mimic shell bone lesions. If there is uncertainty, take multiple views.
- Computed tomography imaging can be utilised to document the extent of bone lesions, particularly in relation to other skeletal structures or the body cavity.
- Generalised loss of bone density may support nutritional disease.

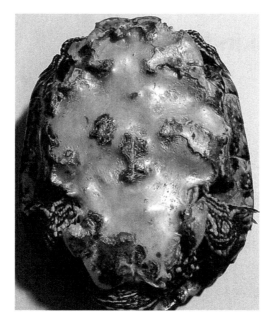

Figure 32.5   Pseudoshell in a Red-eared slider (*Trachemys scripta elegans*).

## Treatment

- Loose scutes should be removed. Often, lesions that appear superficial have progressed into deeper bone. These may require a general anaesthetic if necrotic bone needs to be debrided.
- Appropriate adjustments to husbandry are an important step in any management plan. In some cases, correcting inappropriate husbandry may allow adequate healing with minimal further treatment in animals with focal lesions and otherwise good health.
- The animals' water quality is important and should be maintained within the standard parameters of their natural habitat if possible. Keeping organic loads and bacterial levels low is associated with improved healing. When topping up, use chlorine- and chloramine-free water.
- Deep debriding of extensive lesions will require a general anaesthetic. Usually, the lesion is much deeper than it appears superficially (see Figure 32.5).
- Management of the wound should follow the protocol in the Chapter 18 for contaminated wounds.
- Antimicrobials should be given systemically, on the basis of the culture results.
- Dry docking may be needed for aquatic and semi-aquatic species.

## References

Jackson, C. & Fulton, M. (1970) A turtle colony epizootic apparently of microbial origin. *Journal of Wildlife Diseases*, 6, 466–468.
Wallach, J. (1975) The pathogenesis and etiology of ulcerative shell diseases in turtles. *Journal of Zoo Animal Medicine*, 6, 11–13.

# 33 Skin Ulceration

Skin ulceration is seen occasionally in both terrestrial and aquatic species, though it is more common in the latter. In some cases, it will be accompanied by skin peeling and there is some crossover in investigation of these two syndromes, especially in aquatic species (see Chapter 30).

## Terrestrial species

Primary infection is extremely rare, though it may occur. In one outbreak in a colony that we investigated, spirochaetes were associated with skin lesions. We suspected that cold damp environmental conditions were the primary factors linked to this infection.

A sequel to ulcerative conditions is normally a hypopigmented 'scar' (see Figure 33.1).

Infection secondary to trauma is much more common and may be due to:

- Shell rubbing, especially post-metabolic bone disease with abnormal shell growth and/or incorrect carriage/gait – see Chapter 40 (see also Figure 33.2).
- Obese animals (especially Horsfield's tortoise) or oedematous animals (see Chapters 26 and 37) may suffer skin rubbing against the carapace.
- Rubbing on abrasive surfaces (e.g. concrete), especially if weak or deformities of the shell mean that the animal cannot lift itself on its legs.
- Damage from other animals (especially aggressive biting males – see Chapter 34).
- Thermal damage from heat mats.
- Iatrogenic sloughing following the subcutaneous injection of an irritant substance.

Other differentials may include:

- viral infection (e.g. herpesvirus)
- mycobacterial infection
- neoplasia

*Essentials of Tortoise Medicine and Surgery*, First Edition. John Chitty and Aidan Raftery.
© 2013 John Chitty and Aidan Raftery. Published 2013 by John Wiley & Sons, Ltd.

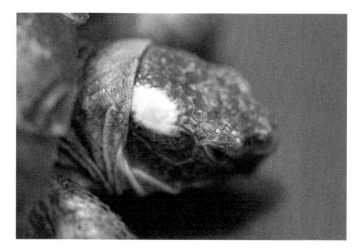

Figure 33.1    A hypopigmented lesion in a Spur-thighed tortoise. Biopsy showed no active inflammation, but the suggestion of prior healed infection.

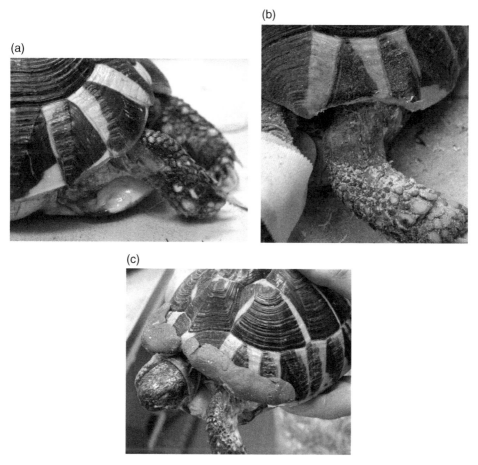

Figure 33.2    Rubbing of the shell on the forelegs (a). Under anaesthesia the shell edges are resected (b) and epoxy applied to the edges (c).

## Investigation

Identification of the underlying cause is the most important step. This relies on a thorough history and clinical examination (see Chapters 2.1 and 4.2), as many of the likely causes may be strongly suspected from the history; owner observation; and distribution of lesions.

The clinical examination should include a full systemic check as well as an examination and description of the lesion(s), as the underlying health may be very important. Investigation of these issues is as described for other generalised problems.

In terms of investigation of the lesion, this will follow a similar course to that described in Chapter 30.

## Sampling

Bacteriological and fungal culture, as well as cytology of infected lesions, should be performed. There is a strong chance of environmental contamination of these lesions, so they should be thoroughly cleaned and debrided before sampling (see Chapter 5.7).

In some cases, deeper biopsy of underlying tissue may be considered more appropriate, both for lesion culture and to determine the underlying cause using histopathology. This is particularly appropriate if the lesions appear unusual; have no obvious underlying cause (especially if present in more than one individual in the same colony); are not responding to therapy based on previous more superficial sampling; or are too heavily contaminated to be sampled.

## Therapy

Appropriate antimicrobials should be selected, on the basis of culture and sensitivity. Topical barrier creams (e.g. silver sulphadiazine cream) are very useful and should be applied after daily cleaning with povidone iodine or F10 SC (1:250 dilution) or chlorhexidine. Superficial lesions may respond to topical therapy alone.

Removal of the underlying cause is vital. Where these are caused by shell rubbing, the animal should be anaesthetised and the portion of shell removed. The cut edge of shell is covered using epoxy resin such that a smooth edge is formed, no longer in direct contact with the skin (see Chapter 40).

## Aquatic species

As in terrestrial species, primary infections are unusual, though opportunistic infections are common. Environmental problems, especially poor water quality, are the most important underlying reasons.

## Underlying causes

- Immunosuppression from underlying disease.
- Poor water quality.
- Chronic stress.
- Trauma from other individuals or from sharp objects within the tank.

## Investigation

Water-quality checks (see Chapter 2.1) and a full evaluation of the environment and stocking rate (including gender ratios) are vital in these cases.

The clinical examination should include a full systemic check as well as examination and description of the lesion(s), as the underlying health may be very important. Investigation of these issues is as described for other generalised problems.

In terms of investigation of the lesion, this will follow a similar course to that described in Chapter 30.

## Sampling

Bacteriological and fungal culture, as well as cytology of lesions, are essential. Bacterial infections appear more common than fungal, though both are possible, and it is impossible to discriminate between these on the visual appearance of lesions.

It is essential to sample lesions after cleaning and debridement – the external layers are only likely to culture environmental contaminants. If in doubt, anaesthetise and biopsy deeper parts of the lesion for culture (see Figure 33.3).

If in doubt, deeper biopsy of underlying tissue may be considered more appropriate both for lesion culture and to determine the underlying cause using histopathology.

(a)

(b)

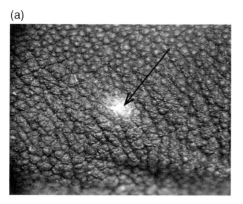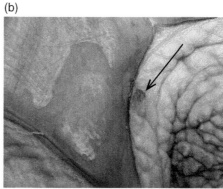

Figure 33.3    (a) A fungal skin infection in a Snake-necked turtle. (b) Bacterial skin ulceration in a Soft-shell turtle. Poor water quality was identified as the underlying cause in both cases.

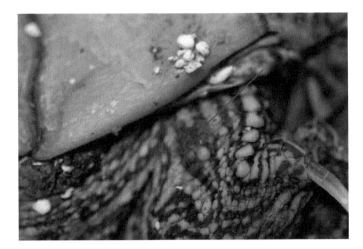

Figure 33.4    In this Red-eared slider, multiple superficial skin abscesses were identified. Biopsy confirmed these to be bacterial. The multiple punctuate appearance of these over most skin areas suggested septicaemic spread.

This is particularly appropriate if the lesions appear unusual; have no obvious underlying cause; are not responding to therapy based on previous more superficial sampling; or are too heavily contaminated to be sampled.

## Therapy

Improvement of water quality and the removal of any other identified underlying causes are mandatory in all cases.

Dry docking (see Chapter 3.3) is generally necessary in semi-aquatic species. For aquatic species, affected individuals must be kept in pristine water conditions with daily water changes. They should be fed using a separate feeding chamber or bowl.

Antimicrobial therapy is also essential. Topical barrier creams (e.g. silver sulphadiazine cream) should be applied after daily cleaning with povidone iodine or F10 SC (1:250 dilution) or chlorhexidine. Superficial lesions may respond to topical therapy alone. Deeper lesions (or cases where there are multiple lesions) will require systemic therapy as well, and this should be based on culture and sensitivity results (see Figure 33.4).

# 34 Soft Tissue Trauma

Soft tissue trauma is relatively common in captive chelonians. First intention healing is rarely possible other than for surgical wounds, due to the relative lack of 'spare' skin and the chronicity of the injuries with which they are often presented.

Common causes of injury are as follows:

- direct trauma – for example, by grass mowers
- bites from dogs, rodents or other tortoises (especially males in the breeding season – in particular, male Hermann's or Horsfield's tortoises) (see Figures 34.1, 34.2 and 34.3)

These wounds should be distinguished from skin ulcers (Chapter 33) – if unsure, they should be investigated for underlying causes as per skin ulceration.

## Pre-surgical preparation

Soft tissue injuries are rarely seen fresh and are often contaminated.

Unless very fresh and clean, it is likely that healing by secondary intention (granulation) will be required. In these cases, it is frequently necessary to delay surgery in order to better prepare the soft tissues.

The exception to this is where emergency haemostasis is required (see Chapter 8.2) or where wounds are very deep and it is felt that delaying surgery will result in excessive suffering to the animal. In these cases, the animal's overall welfare must be considered and if the wounds are too extensive, euthanasia may be considered.

Otherwise, pre-surgical preparation involves the following:

- Fluid therapy is necessary if there is extensive exposure of underlying tissues through skin or shell loss; or if there is obvious haemorrhage; or if the animal appears shocked. The route of fluid therapy and choice of fluids will be dictated by need and by site of damage (see Chapter 5.6). Daily bathing should be carried out as a matter of course.

NB Aquatic species should be dry docked throughout the treatment process – see Chapter 3.3.4.

*Essentials of Tortoise Medicine and Surgery*, First Edition. John Chitty and Aidan Raftery.
© 2013 John Chitty and Aidan Raftery. Published 2013 by John Wiley & Sons, Ltd.

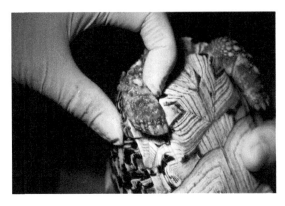

Figure 34.1　Typical rat bites in a Leopard tortoise. Note the bone exposure – nonetheless, with appropriate supportive care for tortoise and wounds, these can heal very well.

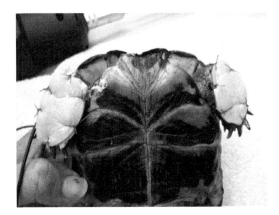

Figure 34.2　A different tortoise after a similar injury. The wounds have been debrided and dressed with a mixture of hydrophilic gel and silver sulphadiazine cream. A Granuflex pad is then sutured over the top. The pads are removed under sedation and wounds cleaned every 2–3 weeks until healed.

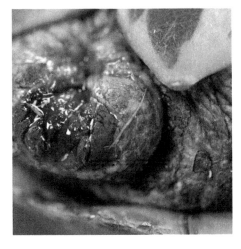

Figure 34.3　A tail bite in a female Hermann's tortoise, following prolonged exposure to a male of the same species.

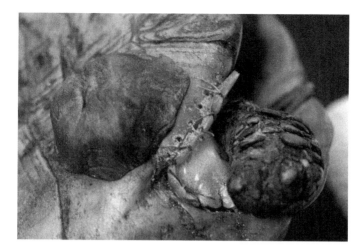

**Figure 34.4** The wound in the axilla has been debrided and covered in a Granuflex dressing (Convatec UK). Note how sutures have been placed through drill holes in the shell, as there was no soft tissue available to use. A sliding prosthesis has been placed to allow the wound to be kept off the ground.

- Systemic antibiosis – ceftazidime is often a good first choice of antibiotic. Fluoroquinolones may also be used, but are not effective against the anaerobic organisms that may be introduced in bite wounds.
- Analgesia – non-steroidal anti-inflammatory drugs (NSAIDs) and/or opiates are very useful (see Chapter 6). If shocked, NSAIDs should be delayed until after fluid therapy has been started. Local anaesthesia can be used by means of a splash block mix of lignocaine and bupivicaine (see Chapter 6.1).
- Regular cleaning – bathing and cleansing of the wound should be carried out daily. Dilute chlorhexidine or povidone iodine or F10SC are all effective agents for wound cleansing.
- Wound covering – silver sulphadiazine cream (Flamazine, Smith & Nephew, Hull, UK) and hydrophilic gels (e.g. Intra Site, Smith & Nephew, Hull, UK) are effective short-term wound coverings for wounds that are difficult to bandage. Either may be used, or a 50:50 mixture of these agents may be applied with, in our experience, good success.
- Bandages – hydrophilic dressings may be applied as bandaging materials, though bandaging tortoise limbs is rarely easy. Dressings should be changed daily due to the need to bathe the animal each day.
- Where the wound is liable to be rubbed/traumatised on the ground, a gliding prosthesis (see Chapter 17) may be applied to the plastron in that region, in order to raise the wound off the ground (see Figure 34.4).

## First intention healing

Wherever possible, wounds should be healed by first intention.

Very small wounds may be repaired using tissue glue (see Chapter 5.8).

Polydioxanone, polyglactin 910 and polyglycolic acid are suitable materials for chelonian skin. They may be left to resorb over 5–6 months or may be removed after 6–8 weeks. If the animal is actively shedding, then wounds should be bathed daily to remove the build-up of shed skin.

The preferred suture pattern is simple interrupted. While some texts advise the use of a horizontal mattress with skin eversion, this may result in excessive tension on the wound, with wound edge necrosis and irritation. Whichever pattern is used, skin tension is critical, as too loose a suture will allow inversion of the wound edges. In some positions, tension-relieving patterns may be employed.

Where the wound is situated adjacent to the shell such that one edge of the wound is formed by the shell, suturing may still be achieved by:

- drilling small suture guide holes in the shell edge (see Figure 34.4), or
- applying epoxy or polymethyl methacrylate to the shell and using this as an anchor for the sutures

In these cases, horizontal mattress sutures are a more appropriate pattern to spread tension and nylon is a more appropriate material.

## Second intention healing

Initially, wounds should be debrided under general anaesthesia.

Silver sulphadiazine cream/hydrophilic gel combinations may be appropriate for long-term use for wounds in places not amenable to bandaging.

However, in most cases of wounds on legs or tails, hydrophilic dressing pads (e.g. Granuflex (Convatec UK, Uxbridge, UK) or Allevyn (Smith & Nephew, Hull, UK)) may be sutured in place. These are relatively hard wearing and require changing only every 2–3 weeks if managed correctly – normally, we will use topical gels (see above) for the first week after injury before debridement under anaesthesia and application of these pads.

Where pads cannot be sutured in place yet bandaging is possible, soft hydrophilic dressings may be applied; for example, Intra Site Conformable (Smith & Nephew, Hull, UK). If contamination remains, silver-impregnated dressings are very useful; for example, Aquacell Ag (Convatec UK, Uxbridge, UK). In these cases, the animal should only be allowed to bath every 3–4 days and the bandage changed at the same time.

Throughout healing, environmental parameters must be kept optimal. Paper is recommended as a substrate, as it is easy to clean on a daily basis. Aquatic species should be dry docked and hibernation is inappropriate during the healing period. Owners should be informed of these needs, as a higher level of commitment and changes to normal husbandry methods may preclude therapy. In addition, healing will often take several months and the cumulative expense may be considerable.

# 35 Swimming Problems

Aquatic or semi-aquatic species may exhibit difficulty swimming. This may be exhibited in a variety of signs.

Reluctance to enter water may manifest as increased basking time, with retention of shell scutes and dysecdysis (see Chapter 30).

Some may show altered buoyancy, with animals either floating or sinking, or alternatively tilting front-to-back or side-to-side when swimming.

In some cases, there may be a complete inability to swim or the animal may only swim in circles.

## Differential diagnoses

These need to be considered by sign, as follows.

1. Reluctance to enter water:
   - Inability to swim or extreme difficulty swimming – see 2 and 3 below.
   - Inhospitable environment – water temperature and/or water quality inappropriate (see Chapter 2.1).
   - The presence of larger, more aggressive animals in the water – this is particularly relevant if animals are fed in water in their normal environment.
2. Altered buoyancy:
   - Solid lesions in the lung fields – abscess or tumour – and including lung rupture (see Figure 35.1).
   - Increased intestinal gas – for example, ileus/gut dysbiosis with gas-producing bacteria (see Chapter 12.2).
   - Increased coelomic cavity gas following injury (especially to a lung) or iatrogenic post-coeloscopy.
   - Focal brain lesion.
   - Abdominal masses – for example, eggs/foreign bodies.

*Essentials of Tortoise Medicine and Surgery*, First Edition. John Chitty and Aidan Raftery.
© 2013 John Chitty and Aidan Raftery. Published 2013 by John Wiley & Sons, Ltd.

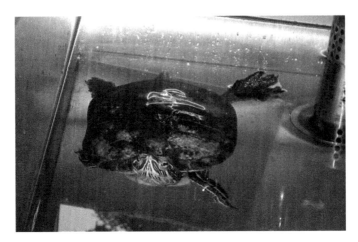

Figure 35.1    A Red-eared slider with right-sided pneumonia: note how the animal tilts to the right. *Source*: Girling, S. and Raiti, P. (eds) (2004) *BSAVA Manual of Reptiles*, 2nd edn. Reproduced with permission of the BSAVA.

3.  Inability to swim, or circling:
    - Neurological disease – space-occupying lesions in the brain, thiamine deficiency, toxins (e.g. lead), aneurysm post-hyperthermia.
    - Hypocalcaemia.
    - Limb damage.

## Investigation

### History

See Chapter 4.2, though important features include: signalment; environmental considerations (including water quality and temperature – see Chapter 2.1); other animals in the environment (species, gender ratios, the size of other individuals); and the nature and timing of the problem.

Owner observations are extremely important in deciding the route of investigation of these problems. Requesting the owners to bring photographs of the environment and, especially, videos of the abnormal behaviour or clinical sign can be extremely useful.

### Examination

A full clinical examination should be performed (see Chapter 4.2).

It can be very useful to fill a large bowl (or tub table; see Figure 35.1) with water in order to observe swimming in the clinic.

## Further tests

- Radiography – dorsoventral and horizontal beam views of the lung fields (lateral and cranio-caudal) are vital, given that lung masses and abdominal foreign bodies are important differentials of these presentations.
- Ultrasonography – of soft tissue masses in the abdomen. Guided biopsy can also be useful.
- Endoscopy of the abdomen or lungs (depending on the presence of lesions) – lesions may also require biopsy for histopathology and/or culture.
- Haematology/biochemistry – if necessary to investigate underlying causes or subclinical disease, or to measure thiamine or lead levels if these are considered to be differentials.

## Therapy

Dependent on cause – see the relevant Chapters in this book.

During therapy, affected animals should be dry docked, with daily swimming sessions – this allows the opportunity to drink as well as enabling monitoring of the condition.

In all cases, environmental correction is important, with maintenance of good water conditions (see Chapter 2.1).

During therapy, animals should be fed in bowls of clean water, separate from the main vivarium. Some need to be in water to feed and defecate, but once this has been performed, they can be placed back in dry dock.

# 36 Swollen Limbs

It is common to see limb swelling in captive chelonians. Initially, it should be determined whether the swelling is in one limb, all limbs or of just fore- or hindquarters.

In other words, is this a generalised or systemic problem or a localised one?

It is then necessary to determine whether the swelling is diffuse or focal. And if focal, is the swelling centred on the joints or in soft tissues or long bones?

In all cases, a thorough history should be taken along with environmental evaluation (see Chapters 2.1 and 4.2) – this is important in assessing issues that may cause immunosuppression. Similarly, while infections are common in all age groups, tumours tend to be in older individuals.

A full clinical examination should always be performed, as more generalised disease may also be present.

The following presentations may be seen.

## Diffuse swelling

### All limbs

See Chapter 26.

### Of either hind- or forelimbs

Consider occlusion of lymph or venous drainage.

It is therefore important to consider the following investigations:

- Imaging of body cavity in that region – radiography or ultrasound to assess the presence of occlusive masses.
- Biopsy – masses may be sampled by fine needle aspiration or cutting needle. Ultrasound guidance may help.

*Essentials of Tortoise Medicine and Surgery*, First Edition. John Chitty and Aidan Raftery.
© 2013 John Chitty and Aidan Raftery. Published 2013 by John Wiley & Sons, Ltd.

- Cytology of aspirated fluid from limbs – however, this is frequently unrewarding, as it is difficult to obtain a representative sample.
- Haematology/biochemistry to consider underlying issues.

## Of one limb

Investigate as for fore-/hind limbs above.

However, localised infections are more common and occlusive lesions more likely to be focal. This places more emphasis on cytology of any aspirated fluid and imaging and biopsy of lesions, and less on haematology/biochemistry as useful tests.

## Focal swelling

### Soft tissue

See Chapter 22. In our experience, the most common soft tissue focal swellings are in or among the phalanges. Diffuse or organised granulomata may cause enlargement of the foot, although soft tissue reactions to gout or inflammatory lesions are also seen. Radiography will show distortion and occasionally resorption of the bones of the foot. Aspiration cytology or core biopsies are of great assistance in these cases. It is rarely possible to remove these lesions surgically. Intra-lesional antimicrobials may be helpful, either with or without systemic antimicrobials and non-steroidal anti-inflammatory drugs. Otherwise, amputation may be indicated (see Chapter 17: see also Figures 36.1, 36.2, 36.3 and 36.4).

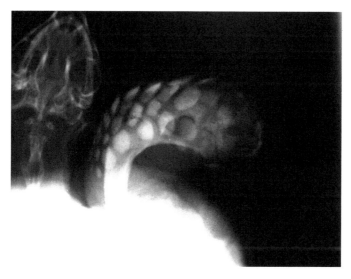

Figure 36.1    Infections in the feet may be erosive.

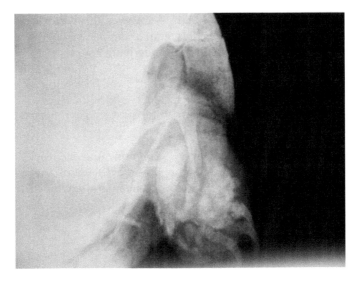

Figure 36.2   Infections in the feet may be calcified. In this case, histopathology suggested an underlying vitamin E deficiency.

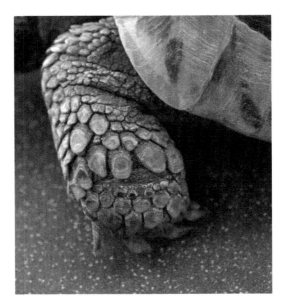

Figure 36.3   Swelling of the forefeet in this Hermann's tortoise was accompanied by weight loss and weakness.

## Bone – swellings or masses on long bones

These are relatively uncommon. Radiography is of most use to view the lesion. These can be biopsied (sedation or anaesthesia are essential) using Jamshidi bone biopsy

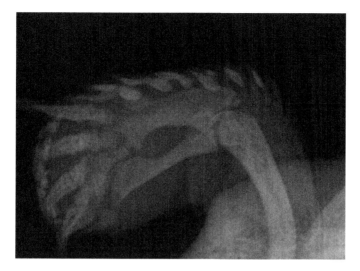

Figure 36.4  Radiographs of the tortoise in 36.3 showed osteolysis and diffuse reaction around the bones. Fine needle aspirates showed uric acid tophi and sepsis, while blood uric acid was markedly elevated. The diagnosis was gout, with a secondary bacterial infection.

needles. See Chapter 17, as one of the most common reasons for an uncommon presentation can be partially callused fractures, with or without infection. Where these lesions cannot be controlled or corrected, amputation may be indicated.

## Joints

It is important to assess all palpable joints, not just those of the limbs (see Figure 36.5), as it is important to assess whether or not the underlying problem is localised or systemic.

For single-joint swelling, consider the following differential diagnoses:

- Osteoarthritis.
- Trauma – cruciate ligament rupture has been reported in the stifle joint of larger tortoises. The cranial draw sign may be present in these cases.
- Septic arthritis.
- Neoplasia.
- Rarely, gout will present with a single joint affected initially.

Differential diagnoses of polyarthritis include the following:

- gout
- septic arthritis
- osteoarthritis

In all cases, radiography of affected joints is required to determine the extent of the changes.

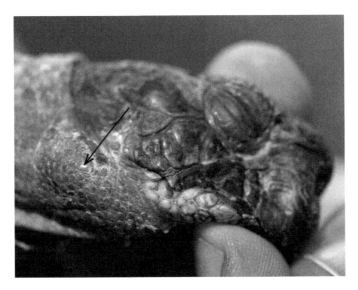

Figure 36.5   It is important to assess all joints and not just those of the limbs. This Spur-thighed tortoise showed swelling of the joints of the hyoid apparatus (swelling under a skin lesion ventral to the ear scale). A fine needle aspirate confirmed septic arthritis.

In very large animals, the joint may be ultrasound scanned or arthroscopically examined.

The most effective test is cytology of joint aspirates – most can be sampled conscious as long as the limb can be restrained outside the shell without undue force. Otherwise, sedation/anaesthesia may be required.

Aspiration is easy, as most tortoise joints are fairly wide and accessible – palpation will confirm the position of more proximal joints; that is, the hip or shoulder.

The skin is prepared aseptically and a 23G needle can be used to access the joint.

Air-dried smears of the aspirate are prepared immediately and a drop of fluid is also placed on a bacteriology swab.

An unstained slide is examined first to check for uric acid crystals.

The finding of gout crystals should be followed by systemic investigation – in particular, haematology/biochemistry looking at renal function and ultrasonography of the kidneys. Endoscopic biopsy of the kidneys may also be considered.

Therapy is unlikely to succeed, as this condition normally represents severe renal failure and gout is extremely painful. If attempted, it should include the following:

- Aggressive fluid therapy (preferably intra-osseous).
- Therapy for underlying disorders, secondary infections and correction of environmental inadequacies.

- Reduction or removal of protein from the diet (if necessary) of herbivorous species. In particular, cat food should not be used for any species, even carnivorous ones.
- Analgesia with non-steroidal anti-inflammatories; for example, meloxicam. These should only be used after instigating fluid therapy, as they may cause further renal damage.
- Allopurinol is advocated by some, though it is rarely effective.

If no gout crystals are present, then the slides should be stained with a trichrome stain; for example 'Diff Quik' (Dade).

These may identify the following:

- Osteoarthritis – typically a proteinaceous (blue) background with some epithelial cells, erythrocytes, heterophils and lymphocytes/ monocytes
- Septic arthritis – a proteinaceous background, with bacteria present. Many degenerate erythrocytes and heterophils monocytes. Typically, heterophils may be toxic in appearance and engulfed bacteria may be present in inflammatory cells. In these cases, bacteriology swabs of joint fluid may be submitted.

**NB** These can give no growth due to the presence of so many inhibitory factors in the fluid.

- Tumour cells.

Therapy of septic arthritis involves the following:

- Systemic antimicrobials – ceftazidime is an excellent first choice, pending positive culture results (unless the morphology of bacteria on cytology suggest that an alternative drug may be more appropriate).
- Joint flushing – hypodermic needles are placed on each side of the joint and the space flushed with saline. When the fluid starts to emerge clear, a small quantity of ceftazidime may be inserted into the joint (see Figure 36.6).
- Systemic non-steroidal anti-inflammatory drugs.
- Correction of underlying husbandry issues.
- If polyarthritis, care must be taken to investigate and locate other abscesses in the body or in the shell (as the spread is likely to be haematogenous). Whole-body radiographs in at least two planes and coelomic ultrasonography should be obtained. The heart should be auscultated using an 8 MHz Doppler device. Lesions on heart valves are associated with harsh murmurs and a poor prognosis. Blood culture may be indicated in these cases (see Chapter 9.3).

Therapy of osteoarthritis involves the following:

- systemic non-steroidal anti-inflammatory drugs
- if a single joint, then it can be flushed and a water-soluble anti-inflammatory injected (e.g. carprofen or meloxicam) intra-articularly (see above)

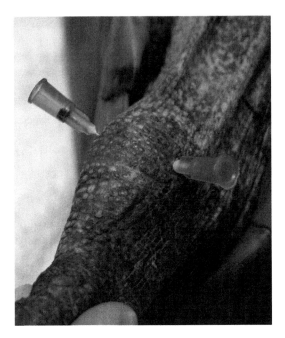

Figure 36.6  A swollen stifle joint. Under sedation, hypodermic needles are placed in the joint on both the lateral and medial sides. Saline is flushed through from one side until only clear fluid emerges from the other. Antibiotic is then instilled into the joint.

In either case, where there is only one joint affected, this may be rested by:

- removing climbing rocks and so on from the vivarium
- restricting the area of movement
- applying a gliding prosthesis of epoxy resin under the shell in that limb's quadrant, to raise it off the ground (see Chapter 17 and Figure 34.4)

In severe cases of joint disease affecting only one limb, amputation may be considered (see Chapter 17).

# 37 Uroliths

Urinary stones present commonly in terrestrial herbivorous species, though some authors feel that *Geochelone sulcata* (the African Spurred tortoise) may be over-represented.

The majority consist of uric acid deposited in the bladder, which coalesces into stones during hibernation or periods of dehydration.

In rare cases, other types of stone (including apatite and struvite) have been recorded, especially in urea-uricotelic species (i.e. carnivorous aquatic or semi-aquatic species).

All should be distinguished from calcified deposits in soft tissues (especially kidneys) that may occur secondary to hypervitaminosis D (see Figure 37.1).

In many cases, these uroliths are asymptomatic and are identified during other investigations – in such cases, they may well represent an indication of a chronic course of disease with reduced hydration and/or urination.

Where clinical signs occur, they are exhibited when the animal tries to pass a stone – these may then become lodged in the pelvic canal or cloaca. In some cases of very large stones, they may be unable to exit the bladder. Blockage is associated with straining and discomfort. Often, urine can still be passed, though complete obstruction may occur – in these cases post-renal renal failure may be a complication.

## Diagnosis

The urolith is often visible in the cloaca. If suspected but not visible, the urolith may be palpated per cloaca, using a finger in larger animals or a blunt probe in smaller ones. Care must be taken not to retropulse the urolith.

Otherwise, the following imaging modalities may be employed:

- radiography (see Figure 37.2)
- ultrasonography – some deposits are radiolucent
- endoscopy of the bladder – sometimes useful for differentiating between uroliths and eggs deposited in the bladder (if not clear on radiography)

*Essentials of Tortoise Medicine and Surgery*, First Edition. John Chitty and Aidan Raftery.
© 2013 John Chitty and Aidan Raftery. Published 2013 by John Wiley & Sons, Ltd.

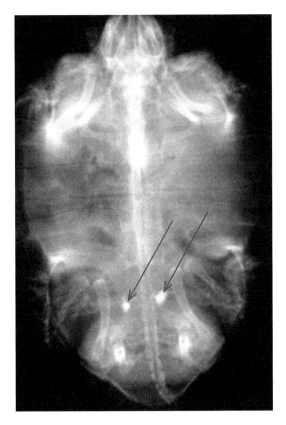

Figure 37.1    Renoliths in a Red-eared slider.

If identified, other investigations are required, as these are a marker of recent/current dehydration/debility:

- full clinical examination (see Chapter 4.2)
- environmental evaluation – in particular, hibernation conditions if recently hibernated (see Chapter 2.1)
- full clinical history – if possible, pre-hibernation weight, management and so on (see Chapter 4.2)
- haematology/biochemistry (see Chapter 9.1)

Once removed, urate deposits are readily identified: normally these stones are rough, white and crumble relatively easily. Some crumbled material may be placed on a microscope slide in a drop of water and urate crystals are easily identified. Stones of abnormal appearance should be submitted to a commercial laboratory for identification.

## Therapy

If there are no associated signs, then specific therapy may not be needed, though it may be felt that these will be likely to grow and so should be removed once the animal's major clinical issues are stabilised or resolved. However, any other clinical

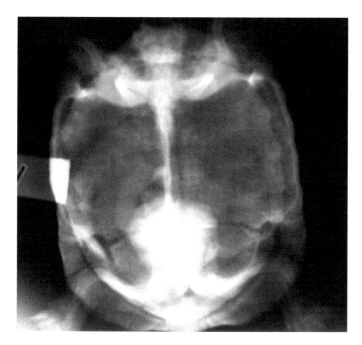

Figure 37.2    A large urolith in a tortoise.

problems should be addressed. The tortoise should be encouraged to drink (regular daily or twice daily bathing, as well as spraying the food with water) and may be fed dandelion to encourage diuresis. Stone size and position should be monitored at intervals.

Where identified, non-urate deposits may require specific dietary management, dependent on type.

If the urolith is lodged in the cloaca, these deposits can normally be removed relatively easily under sedation/anaesthesia. Larger stones may be broken down *in situ*, or the cloacal opening may require enlargement via a ventral incision. There is often a cloacitis caused by the rough material, which can be managed with local cleaning and application of mouth ulcer gels.

If the urolith is lodged in the bladder, the procedure can be considerably more difficult. Under anaesthesia, it may be possible to physically break down and remove endoscopically piecemeal per cloaca. Alternatively, ultrasonic lithotripsy under endoscopic guidance may be possible. Failing this, cystotomy (via plastron osteotomy) may be required (see Chapter 8.3).

## Prevention

Maintenance of adequate hydration via diet and access to regular bathing is generally adequate. In particular, good husbandry practice around hibernation/aestivation periods will help.

# 38 Vomiting and Regurgitation

It is very difficult to distinguish between vomiting and regurgitation in Chelonia, so here they will be considered as a single entity for the purposes of clinical investigation.

This is an unusual presentation – the most common exhibition of vomition is normally iatrogenic after stomach tubing. However, where it is seen it can be an indicator of severe disease, especially if occurring frequently and if the animal appears unwell. Such cases should be seen as a matter of urgency.

Otherwise, the animal will rarely perform this action in front of the clinician, so a good history is vital (see Chapters 2.1 and 4.2).

In particular, the following should be assessed:

- Husbandry/environment.
- Mixing with other tortoises and period owned.
- The timing of vomition after eating.
- How long and how often it occurred (if one-off, the animal is eating and appears well on clinical examination, with negative results on faecal parasitology, then further observation may be all that is required at that stage).
- Content of vomitus:
  - o Is it foamy in appearance?
  - o Food – if so, is it digested or undigested?
  - o Is blood present? If so, is it digested or undigested?
  - o Colour?
- Is the animal anorexic?
- Faecal output and appearance.
- Possibility of foreign body ingestion.

Differentials include the following:

- generalised gut disease
- endoparasitism
- gastritis – bacterial, fungal or parasitic
- focal oesophageal mass or lesion

*Essentials of Tortoise Medicine and Surgery*, First Edition. John Chitty and Aidan Raftery.
© 2013 John Chitty and Aidan Raftery. Published 2013 by John Wiley & Sons, Ltd.

- foreign body
- toxicity – including rhododendron

## Diagnostic investigation

A full clinical examination (see Chapter 4.2) is required, in particular to assess the body condition, the mucous membrane colour and the appearance of the pharynx.

The pre-femoral fossae may be palpated while the tortoise is gently rocked side-to-side. Large solid objects may be detected – for example, a stone, eggs or uroliths (see Figure 38.1).

Further investigation should include the following:

- Faecal parasitology is required. Where a sample cannot be obtained, cloacal washes can be used (see Chapter 9.3).
- If available, a fresh sample of vomitus should be examined for cytology and parasites. It can also be submitted for bacteriology/sensitivity.
- A haematology and biochemistry screen is mandatory in such cases.

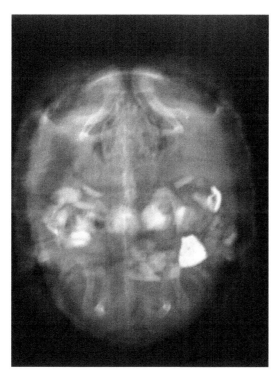

Figure 38.1    Many tortoises will contain large numbers of stones in the gut. These may be retained for long periods – even years – and can be very misleading in these cases, as they are usually of no clinical significance.

- Radiography, including plain views and barium studies:
  - barium should be tube fed as a liquid (10 ml/kg)
  - dorso-ventral and lateral (horizontal beam) radiographs should be taken immediately and then at 2 hourly intervals over 24–96 hours, depending on the gut transit time
- Endoscopy of stomach and stomach wash for cytology/culture. Focal lesions in the oesophagus or stomach may be sampled for cytology using a brush technique. Pinch biopsies are risky, as full-thickness sampling could well lead to coelomitis. NB This should be performed BEFORE barium study!
- Ultrasonography may reveal some detail of the stomach wall, but is rarely of much help in these cases. CT or MRI (if available) may be more appropriate.

## Therapy

As ever, any underlying issues should be addressed and corrected:

- Foreign bodies will probably require coelotomy and surgical removal (Chapter 8.3.2), though endoscopic removal may be contemplated for smooth gastric foreign bodies (Chapter 7.3).
- Anti-emetics (e.g. maropitant) are not indicated.
- Prokinetics (e.g. metoclopramide) are often used in cases of ileus/gastric stasis or bloat where there is no indication of an obstructive foreign body.
- Intracoelomic fluids should be used with care unless it is clear that there is no gross coelomic pathology. Ideally, fluids should be given intra-osseously in these cases.
- In cases of gastritis or gastric ulceration, sucralfate suspension may be a useful adjunctive therapy.
- Anti-microbial and anti-parasitic agents may be used where indicated by results of diagnostic testing.
- In cases of toxicoses, where the toxin is still in the stomach, gastric lavage or endoscopic removal under sedation or anaesthesia may be attempted. In addition, the animal should be given fluid, anti-bacterial and biological support. After removal, coating agents (see above) and adsorbents (e.g. activated charcoal) may be used. However, in such cases it is good to obtain specific advice (see Appendix 3).

# 39 Metabolic Bone Diseases

There are many types of metabolic bone disease. The veterinary surgeon must identify what type of metabolic bone disease is present. The most common metabolic bone disease diagnosed in chelonians is nutritional secondary hyperparathyroidism, also referred to as nutritional metabolic bone disease. Renal secondary hyperparathyroidism is the second most common type of metabolic bone disease seen in chelonians. It is also sometimes called renal metabolic bone disease. Other metabolic diseases of bone are rare in chelonians.

## Nutritional secondary hyperparathyroidism

### Causes

- A dietary deficiency in calcium.
- Inadequate exposure to the correct band of ultraviolet light in the basking zone.
- Excess dietary phosphorus.
- Low temperatures, which impair digestion.
- Unnatural diets, causing an excessively rapid growth rate (high-protein diets are often anecdotally associated with rapid growth, but other factors probably also influence growth rate). See nutrition in Chapter 2.1, and see also Figure 39.1.

### Symptoms

- Most commonly seen in juveniles, where the more rapid growth rate will exacerbate the signs.
- The shell – especially the plastron – becomes flexible. In severe cases, it can be very soft, with the animal unable to bear weight.
- The jaw may be deformed and soft.
- Posterior paresis may be present.

*Essentials of Tortoise Medicine and Surgery*, First Edition. John Chitty and Aidan Raftery.
© 2013 John Chitty and Aidan Raftery. Published 2013 by John Wiley & Sons, Ltd.

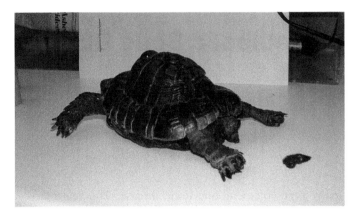

Figure 39.1    A *Testudo graeca* with a chronically deformed shell.

## Diagnostic tests

- Radiography – however, radiography is not a sensitive diagnostic test for early metabolic bone disease. Evaluation can be subjective. Digital radiography has removed some of the technical errors by improving image quality, reducing noise, removing technical artefacts and optimising contrast:
  - o   generalised decreased bone density
  - o   cortical thinning of the long bones
  - o   pathological fractures, both old healed and recent
  - o   angular deformities of the long bones
  - o   deformities of the carapace, plastron and their joining bridges
  - o   opacity of the bones of the pectoral and pelvic girdles
- Environment, diet and physical examination findings will raise suspicion of a metabolic bone disease.
- A haematology and biochemistry screen will give information about concurrent disease that will affect the treatment plan (see Chapter 9.1).
- Total calcium and phosphorus values and their ratio. A calcium:phosphorus ratio less than 1:1 will raise the suspicion of NMBD, especially if there is a hypocalcaemia and a hyperphosphatemia. Total calcium levels are normal in most cases.
- Ionised calcium is reduced only in severe cases. It should be noted that post-sampling changes and minor haemolysis will result in lowering of ionised calcium readings and also a rise in phosphate levels. Testing on the spot gives the most accurate results – or if not available, then submit a sample spun in a heparin gel tube.
- Calcidiol (25-hydroxycholecalciferol) blood levels (Eatwell 2008).

## Treatment

- Correct any environmental and dietary deficiencies. This is the most important treatment step.

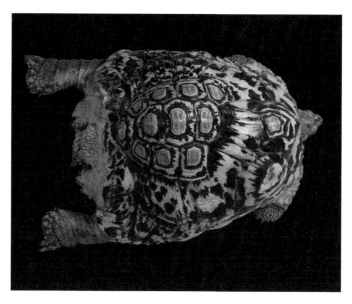

Figure 39.2   A Leopard tortoise with a severely deformed carapace caused by nutritional secondary hyperparathyroidism when it was a juvenile.

- Oral calcium supplementation (see Appendix 1) – parenteral calcium is rarely indicated and is not without risk, as well as being painful. In other reptiles, it has been used to treat hypocalcaemic tetany, but this is a rare sign in chelonians.
- Calcitonin is commonly used for the treatment of metabolic disease in lizards. There is a paucity of research and little anecdotal experience on its use in chelonians.

## Prognosis

Most cases seen are chronic and respond over a period of weeks to months to correction of the husbandry deficits and calcium supplementation. If there is renal damage and if the shell is very soft, then the prognosis should be guarded (see Figure 39.2).

# Renal secondary hyperparathyroidism

## Causes

- Chronic renal disease will eventually cause hyperparathyroidism.
- Nutritional secondary hyperparathyroidism will lead to renal damage.

## Symptoms

- Usually, the symptoms are non-specific: emaciated, dehydrated, anorexic, depressed and weak.
- Symptoms listed under nutritional secondary hyperparathyroidism are also seen.

## Diagnostic tests

- Hyperphosphatemia as a result of phosphate retention.
- Low calcidiol (25-hydroxycholecalciferol), due to interference with its production in the kidneys.
- Non-regenerative anaemia.
- Dehydration (which may mask the anaemia).
- Uric acid levels are an unreliable indicator of renal pathology (see Chapter 9.1).
- Radiographs may reveal renomegaly, uroliths and changes associated with gout. The skeletal changes listed under nutritional secondary hyperparathyroidism may also be seen.
- Ultrasound can be used to evaluate the kidneys.
- Renal biopsies can give additional information on the pathology in the kidney and on the prognosis, but due to the chelonian anatomy are difficult to collect. If there is a suspicion of renal pathology during a coeliotomy, then a renal biopsy can be easily collected. Otherwise, a biopsy can be collected by coelioscopy; however, the risks of the procedure in an individual with advanced renal disease need to be considered.

## Treatment

- Fluid therapy is vital, especially where there is dehydration and hyperuricaemia.
- Calcium supplementation. However, if there is raised phosphate, then raising calcium before reducing blood phosphate levels may result in soft tissue mineralisation.
- Environment and diet need to be optimum for recovery.
- Once hydrated, nutritional support will be required unless eating (see Chapter 5.4.1).
- Allopurinol has been found helpful anecdotally (see Appendix 1).

## Prognosis

A very soft shell with exudative fluid between the scutes and the bone plates carries a grave prognosis. Uric acid levels above 1000 µmol/l carries a guarded prognosis, but if above 2000 µmol/l recovery is unlikely and euthanasia should be considered. Levels of uric acid levels below 1000 µmol/l carry a reasonable prognosis and most will respond to aggressive treatment. Renal biopsies can help with prognosis (see above).

## Reference

Eatwell, K. (2008) Plasma concentrations of 25-hydroxycholecalciferol in 22 captive tortoises (*Testudo* species). *Veterinary Record*, **162**(11), 342–345.

# 40 Shell Deformities

Deformed shells often do not cause any obvious clinical signs in the animal. However, sometimes the shape of the shell is such that it rubs on the skin as the tortoise is walking, eventually leading to ulceration of the skin (see Chapter 33). Shell abnormalities can also affect the anatomical position and range of movement of the legs, thus affecting ambulation. This can result in abnormal wear on the toes and the nails, which in severe cases may result in areas of pododermitis, where there is excessive wear and overgrowth of the nails on the areas receiving reduced wear.

## Shell distortion

- Healed fractures may in themselves cause distortion and they are likely to result in increasing deformation as the animal grows.
- Congenital deformities may be a result of inappropriate incubation.
- Metabolic bone diseases can cause softening of the shell, which results in deformities. These deformities are then exacerbated as the animal grows.

## Shell flattening

This is normal in some species; for example, the pancake tortoise. However, pathological flattening of the carapace can occur in juvenile tortoises secondary to:

- metabolic bone diseases
- excessive growth usually due to incorrect diet
- trauma

## Shell pyramiding

Pyramiding is the development of symmetrical pyramid-shaped bony growths of the carapace. In some species – for example, *Geochelone elegans* (the Indian Star tortoise) and the three tortoises from the genus *Psammobates* (the Geometric tortoise, the Serrated star tortoise and the African Tent tortoise) – pyramiding

*Essentials of Tortoise Medicine and Surgery*, First Edition. John Chitty and Aidan Raftery.
© 2013 John Chitty and Aidan Raftery. Published 2013 by John Wiley & Sons, Ltd.

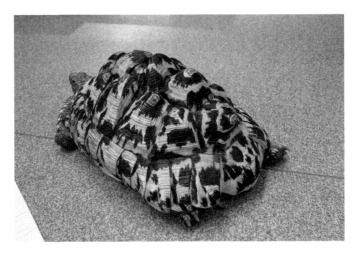

Figure 40.1   A Leopard tortoise with pyramiding.

of the carapace is regarded as normal. However, in most species it is regarded as pathological (see Figure 40.1).

Pyramiding of the shell is most common in herbivorous tortoises, with *Geochelone sulcata*, the African Spur-thighed tortoise, being the most commonly affected species presented.

There are various theories as to the cause of pyramiding. One study showed a relationship between low humidity and pyramiding. An excessive intake of dietary protein and rapid growth rates have also been suggested as possible causes.

## Shell discoloration/changes to scute appearance

- Septicaemia can cause a pinkish discoloration of the plastron, which will blanche with digital pressure (see Figure 33.1).
- Coloured substrates can discolour the plastron.
- Food substances such as strawberries and beetroot will cause discoloration of the shell and skin.
- Healed shell fractures usually have different pigmentation to the adjoining normal shell (see Figure 40.2).
- Aquatic and semi-aquatic chelonians are often presented with algae growing on the carapace. This does not cause any obvious problems for the animal. Poor water quality is more likely to result in excessive algae growth. Lack of normal basking behaviour will also predispose to excessive algae growth. This may indicate an underlying problem needing investigation, or the animal may not be provided with an effective basking area, where the drying of the shell, together with heat and the UV radiation, would reduce algae growth (see Figure 40.3).
- Areas of exposed dermal bone appear white or greyish in colour.
- Burn-damaged areas of shell can sometimes be blackened; however, more commonly there is no visual change until the damaged scutes slough.

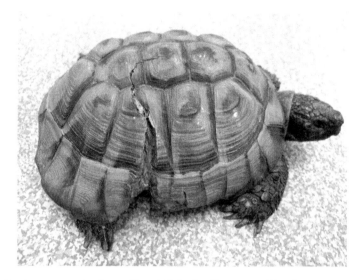

Figure 40.2    A carapace fracture with a deficit after five years of healing.

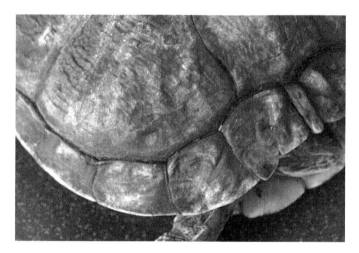

Figure 40.3    Algae growing on the carapace of a Red-eared slider (*Trachemys scripta elegans*).

- Abrasions of the scutes can be seen on the plastron if there is abnormal ambulation resulting in rubbing; also, those kept on a concrete surface or similar will have increased wear on the scutes of the plastron. This is rarely of any consequence except for cosmetic changes.
- When a male is kept with a female, repeated copulation attempts will often cause abrasion of the scutes of the carapace. This only happens as the female cannot escape from the male. They should be separated.
- Environments with concrete sides or large rocks to squeeze past will cause wear to the sides of the carapace, which should not cause any problems unless it is excessive.

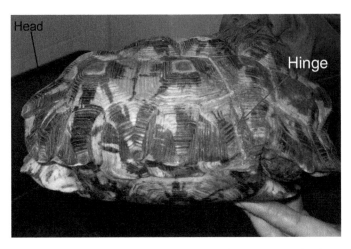

Figure 40.4    Note the caudal hinge in the carapace in Speke's hinge-back tortoise (*Kinixys spekii*).

## Soft shell

- Tortoises hatch with relatively soft shells, which – with correct diet and environmental conditions – harden gradually over the first 6–12 months.
- Soft-shelled turtles should be identified so that their normal anatomy is not misidentified as a pathological change.
- Many species have plastron hinges.
- The Hinge-backs (*Kinixys* species) have a caudal carapacial hinge (see Figure 40.4).
- *Testudo* species (except for *Testudo horsfieldi*, Horsfield's tortoise), have some plastron mobility between the abdominal and femoral scutes (see Figure 1.4.2).
- Generalised soft shell is most commonly due to nutritional metabolic bone disease. The femoral and anal scutes of the plastron are affected first in most species, and are usually the worst-affected area of the shell in advanced cases.
- Extreme softening of the shell, with fluid accumulating between the scutes and the bone, is a very poor prognostic indicator. There is generally advanced metabolic bone disease, together with organ failure and/or septicaemia.

# Appendix 1
## Formulary

The following is a selection of drug doses for use in Chelonia as described in the text.

It is not intended to be a complete list of drugs to be used in these species, nor is it intended as anything other than a practical guide. Most lack pharmacokinetic or dynamic evaluation in these species, but have gained use through use in clinical practice and so are often cited in texts. For more complete drug listings and referencing, the reader is advised to refer to:

- Carpenter, J.W. (2012) *Exotic Animal Formulary*, 4th edn, Elsevier, Amsterdam.

Most of these drugs are not licensed for use in Chelonia in the UK. Readers are strongly advised to be familiar with prescribing legislation in their own country and to comply with this *vis-à-vis* choice of drugs, manner of supply and supply of appropriate warning/safety information.

Anaesthetic/sedative doses are included in Chapter 6.

| Type of drug | Drug name | Dose and route | Comments |
|---|---|---|---|
| Anti-bacterial | Amikacin | 5 mg/kg im: then 2.5 mg/kg im q3d | Potentially nephrotoxic. Use with care in dehydrated animals and provide fluid support. Due to the presence (though unproven clinical relevance) of the renal portal system, some authorities recommend that aminoglycosides are only injected in the cranial half of the body. |
| | Ceftazidime | 20 mg/kg im q3d | |
| | Doxycycline | 10 mg/kg po q24h 50 mg/kg weekly im* | 'Vibravenos' – Pfizer: human depot preparation. |

*(Continued)*

*Essentials of Tortoise Medicine and Surgery*, First Edition. John Chitty and Aidan Raftery.
© 2013 John Chitty and Aidan Raftery. Published 2013 by John Wiley & Sons, Ltd.

| Type of drug | Drug name | Dose and route | Comments |
|---|---|---|---|
| | Enrofloxacin | 5–10 mg/kg im/po q24h | **NB** Licensed in the UK. Can be very tissue irritant and can cause hypersalivation and anorexia by injection, so need to switch to oral use as soon as it is felt that animal can adequately metabolise the drug by this route. Always use 2.5% injectable preparation. |
| | Marbofloxacin | 10 mg/kg q48h im 5 mg/kg q24h im | Not tissue irritant. |
| | Metronidazole | 12.5–40 mg/kg q24h | Should be used with care because of effects on gut fauna. Use for as short a course as possible – maximum 5–7 day course. Overdosage may cause neurological signs – see Appendix 3. |
| | Trimethoprim-sulphonamide | 20–30 mg/kg po/im q24h | Should be used with care in dehydration, as may cause crystalluria. |
| Anti-fungal | Itraconazole | 5 mg/kg po q24h | Accurate dosing important – some authorities feel that it may be potentially toxic in chelonia, as adverse effects have been observed in other reptile groups. Monitoring of blood parameters (especially liver) useful in long-term usage (see Chapter 9.1). |
| | Nystatin | 100 000 IU/kg po q24h | Enteric yeast infection. NOT absorbed from the gut. |
| | Terbinafine | 15 mg/kg po q24h | |
| | Voriconazole | 10 mg/kg po q24h | May be safer than itraconazole. |
| Anti-viral | Acyclovir | 80 mg/kg tid po 80 mh/kg q72h | Efficacy not proven in chelonians. Reported to cause renal damage (Schumacher 1996; McArthur et al. 2004). |
| Anti-parasitic | | | **IVERMECTIN MUST NOT BE USED!** |
| | Cypermethrin/ piperonyl butoxide | | F10 (Health & Hygiene Pty) combined preparation may be used in the treatment of myiasis as a localised wash or flush (provided that lesions do not enter the coelomic cavity or lungs). |

| Type of drug | Drug name | Dose and route | Comments |
|---|---|---|---|
| | Emodepsid/ praziquantel | 2 ml/kg percutaneously | 'Profender' (Bayer) shown to be effective against nematodes and cestodes. |
| | Fenbendazole | 50 mg/kg q24h×3 | Benzimidazoles may cause blood dyscrasias and immunosuppression. |
| | | | **NB** Fenbendazole metabolised to oxfendazole for effect-animal must be in optimal condition to rely on its efficacy: for this reason, it is unlikely to be effective in single doses. |
| | Levamisole | 5–20 mg/kg po/im once | Doubts over its efficacy in reptiles. |
| | Metronidazole | 12.5–40 mg/kg q24h | Should be used with care because of effects on gut fauna. Use for as short a course as possible. |
| | Oxfendazole | 68 mg/kg po | Benzimidazoles may cause blood dyscrasias and immunosuppression. |
| | Permethrin | | Topical use – direct application to ectoparasites. |
| | Praziquantel | 5–10 mg/kg im/po Repeat in 14 days | |
| | Toltrazuril | 15 mg/kg po eod×3 | |
| | Ponazuril | 20 mg/kg q24h for 28 days PO | Coccidiosis. |
| Analgesic agents | Local anaesthetic agents | | May be used for local analgesia. |
| | Buprenorphine | 0.02–0.2 mg/kg im q12h | |
| | Morphine | 0.05–4 mg/kg im or sc q12–24 h | |
| | | 0.1– 0.2 mg/kg im or iv q24–48 h | |
| | Tramadol | 10 mg/kg po q96h; 10 mg/kg sc q12–48 h | Doses evaluated in red-eared sliders. Respiratory depression has been noted (Souza and Cox 2011). |
| Anti-inflammatory drugs | Carprofen | 1–4 mg/kg im q24–72 h | Mosley (2011). |

(Continued)

| Type of drug | Drug name | Dose and route | Comments |
|---|---|---|---|
| | Meloxicam | 0.1–0.5 mg/kg po/ im q24h | Evaluated in the green iguana. Doses at the higher end of the range produced mild unexplained plasma biochemistry changes, though no clinical adverse effects were noted (Mosley 2011). |
| Nebulisation agents | Acetyl cysteine | 22 mg/ml sterile water | |
| | F10 SC | | Dilute 1:250. |
| | Hypertonic saline | | |
| Miscellaneous drugs | Allopurinol | 50 mg/kg po q24h | |
| | Atenolol | 7 mg/kg im | |
| | Atropine | 0.02–0.04 mg/kg im q12–24 h | Toxicoses. 0.4 mg/kg used in organophosphate/carbamate toxicity. |
| | B-vitamin complex | 10 mg/kg im | May be used as an appetite stimulant. |
| | Calcium borogluconate | 400 mg/kg po q12h | |
| | Calcium gluconate | 10–200 mg/kg im/iv | Dose dependent on need. |
| | Cholestyramine gel | 5 ml/kg po | |
| | Cisapride | 2 mg/kg po q24h | |
| | Diazepam | 2.5 mg/kg im/iv | Use as required for seizures. |
| | Furosemide | 5 mg/kg im q24h | |
| | Nandrolone laurate | 1 mg/kg im q7–14d | May be used as an appetite stimulant. |
| | Metoclopramide | 5–10 mg/kg im/po q24h | Efficacy not proven in reptiles; however, anecdotal reports indicate that it may be useful. |
| | Oxytocin | 5–10 IU/kg im | |
| | Proligestone | 20 mg/kg im | Proposed for follicular stasis. |
| | Propranolol | 1 mg/kg im | |
| | Silybin | 0.4 g/kg po q24h | Milk thistle extract, medical grade. Marketed in the UK as Samylin (Vet Plus). |
| | Sodium calcium edetate | 50 mg/kg im q48h | Heavy metal toxicity. |

| Type of drug | Drug name | Dose and route | Comments |
|---|---|---|---|
| | Sucralfate | 0.5–1.0 g/kg po q24h | |
| | Vitamin B1 (thiamine) | 25 mg/kg im/po q 24h | |
| | Vitamin K1 | 2.5 mg/kg im q24h | Coumarol toxicity. |
| Topical agents | Acyclovir | | Topical agent may be used for viral conjunctivitis/skin lesions. |
| | Fusidic acid | | Ophthalmic and dermal preparations available. Avoid steroid-containing preparations. |
| | Ketorolac | | Ocular NSAID. |
| | Ofloxacin | | Ocular antibiotic. |
| | Prednisolone | | Ocular preparation available. Should only be used where there is no evidence of infection or corneal ulceration. Should monitor for adverse effects of systemic absorption. |
| | Silver sulphadiazine | | Used as anti-bacterial barrier cream for use on skin/shell. |
| | TRIS-EDTA solutions | | May be used in multi-resistant bacterial infections to increase sensitivity to anti-bacterials. |

# References

McArthur, S., Wilkinson, R. and Meyer, J. (2004) *Medicine and Surgery of Tortoises and Turtles*. Blackwell, Oxford.

Mosley, C. (2011) Pain and nociception in reptiles. *Veterinary Clinics of North America: Exotic Animal Practice*, **14**, 45–60.

Schumacher, J. (1996) Viral diseases. In: *Reptile Medicine and Surgery* (ed. D.R. Mader), pp. 224–234. Saunders, St Louis, MO.

Souza, M.J. and Cox, S.K. (2011) Tramadol use in zoologic medicine. *Veterinary Clinics of North America: Exotic Animal Practice*, **14**, 117–130.

# Appendix 2
## Haematological Normals

Care must always be taken when using tables of 'normals', as there is always variance between laboratories. These figures, therefore, must be taken as guidance only and should not be used instead of a laboratory's own normal values.

Use of ISIS normals must always be done in the knowledge that this database, while being very large, also includes sick animals.

| Parameter | *Testudo* spp. | Leopard tortoise | Sulcata | Red-eared Slider | Red-footed tortoise |
|---|---|---|---|---|---|
| PCV (l/l) | 0.32–0.45 (summer 0.2–0.35) | 0.17–0.29 | 0.19–0.37 | 0.25–0.33 | 0.19–0.35 |
| RBC ($10^{12}$/l) | 0.55– 1.25 (summer 0.46–0.87) | 0.6–1.2 | 0.6–1.1 | 0.3–0.8 | 0.5–2.1 |
| Hb (g/dl) | 6.1–13.0 | 2.1–18.5 | 7.3–14.5 | 8.0 | 6.9–8.1 |
| MCV (fl) | 350–490 | 302–526 | 255–513 | 310–1000 | 250–520 |
| MCH (pg) | 90–160 | 109–157 | 109–157 | 95–308 | 118–154 |
| MCHC (g/dl) | 25.0–35.0 | 24–42 | 24–48 | 25.0–35.0 | 28.8–32.4 |
| Total white cell count ($10^9$/l) | 1.0–5.0 | 3.1–13.3 | 1.1–13.3 | 1.0–5.0 | 3.7–11.9 |
| Heterophil ($10^9$/l) | 0.5–3.0 | 0.2–3.0 | 0.2–9.6 | 0.5–3.0 | 1.0–6.35 |
| Lymphocyte ($10^9$/l) | 0.5–1.5 | 0.2–2.5 | 0.1–3.5 | 0.5–1.5 | 0.2–9.8 |
| Monocyte ($10^9$/l) | 0–0.2 | 0–1.0 | 0–1.0 | 0–0.2 | 0–0.76 |
| Eosinophil ($10^9$/l) | 0–0.2 | 0–0.37 | 0–0.2 | 0–0.2 | 0–0.2 |
| Basophil ($10^9$/l) | 0–0.7 | 0–0.4 | 0–0.7 | 0–0.7 | 0–0.7 |
| ALKP (IU/l) | 10–94 | 54–272 | 12–63 | 81–343 | <183 |
| AST (IU/l) | 15–210 | 35–344 | 34–400 | <420 | <600 |

*Essentials of Tortoise Medicine and Surgery*, First Edition. John Chitty and Aidan Raftery.
© 2013 John Chitty and Aidan Raftery. Published 2013 by John Wiley & Sons, Ltd.

| Parameter | *Testudo* spp. | Leopard tortoise | Sulcata | Red-eared Slider | Red-footed tortoise |
|---|---|---|---|---|---|
| Bile acids | <50 | | | | |
| Urea (mmol/l) | <2.1 | <2.1 | <2.1 | <2.1 | <2.1 |
| Uric acid (μmol/l) | 35–450 | 30–500 | 125–625 | 100–400 | 35–450 |
| Cholesterol (mmol/l) | 1.0–4.5 | 0.93–6.1 | 1.5–10.2 | | 1.2–7.36 |
| Glucose (mmol/l) | 0.5–2.2 (spring 6.4–22) | 0.83–11.49 | 3.0–15.3 | 1.1–6.3 | 0.9–9.5 |
| Calcium (mmol/l) | 1.65–3.30 | 2.28–5.3 | 1.65–4.8 | 3.49–3.73 | 2.28–3.95 |
| Phosphate (mmol/l) | 0.48–1.81 | 0.55–2.13 | 0.48–2.52 | 1.19–1.39 | 0.55–1.87 |
| Potassium (mmol/l) | 3.9–4.8 | 4.9–7.5 | 3.6–7.6 | 4.3–8.3 | 4.2–6.8 |
| Sodium (mmol/l) | 130–150 | 125–154 | 125–150 | 133–140 | 116–133 |
| Total protein (g/l) | 23.0–43.0 | 16–64 | 23–50 | 28–66 | 29–72 |
| Albumin (g/l) | 13.0–26.0 | 10–26 | 13–20 | 8–25 | 10–28 |
| Globulin (g/l) | 14.0–29.0 | 10–40 | 14–29 | 12–37 | 17–53 |

## Further reading

CTDS Ltd, Leeds, UK – laboratory normal.

Carpenter, J.W. (2005) *Exotic Animal Formulary*, 3rd edn, Elsevier, Amsterdam.

Girling, S.J. & Raiti, P. (eds) (2004) *BSAVA Manual of Reptiles*, 2nd edn, BSAVA, Quedgeley, UK.

International Species Information System ('ISIS') reference ranges for physiological values in captive wildlife (2002).

# Appendix 3
## Toxicoses

Toxicoses occur rarely in Chelonia. Nonetheless, the clinician does need to be aware of them and of how to recognise them.

In most cases, signs are generalised and non-specific. A good history, therefore, is essential. With respect to toxic plants, a knowledge of botany is required, along with a good reference guide, as captive chelonians may encounter potentially toxic plants both in the home and growing wild in the garden. If in doubt, it is recommended that owners bring some of the flowers and leaves of the ingested plant(s) to the consultation.

The following is a suggested reference guide:

- Frohne, P. & Pfänder, H.J. (2004) *Poisonous Plants*, 2nd edn, Manson, London.

Many plants have been suggested as toxic to tortoises – proven in very few cases and often extrapolated from other species; nonetheless, it is better to be safe than sorry, and the following provides a list of household plants best kept away from tortoises (for more details, see the Tortoise Trust website: http://www.tortoisetrust.org/).

### Plants suspected to be toxic to tortoises

NB Not all parts of plants are toxic, or they may vary in toxicity – for example, the bulb is the most toxic part of the Amaryllis plant. In general, flowers are the least toxic parts of the plants.

Amaryllis (*Amaryllis* spp.)
Arrowhead plant, Nephthytis (*Syngonium podophyllum*)
Asparagus fern (*Asparagus setaceus plumosus*)
Azalea (*Rhododendron occidentale*)
Bird of paradise (*Poinciana gilliesii*)
Bittersweet (*Solanum dulcamara*)
Boston ivy (*Parthenocissus quinquefolia*)
Caladium (*Caladium* sp.)
Chenille plant (*Acalypha hispida*)
Christmas rose (*Helleborus niger* L.)

*Essentials of Tortoise Medicine and Surgery*, First Edition. John Chitty and Aidan Raftery.
© 2013 John Chitty and Aidan Raftery. Published 2013 by John Wiley & Sons, Ltd.

Chrysanthemum (*Chrysanthemum* sp.)
Creeping Charlie, Ground ivy (*Glechoma hederacea*)
Creeping fig (*Ficus*)
Croton (*Codiaeum variegatum*)
Crown of thorns (*Euphorbia milii*)
Dumbcane (*Dieffenbachia seguine*)
Emerald duke (*Philodendron hastatum*)
English ivy (*Hedera helix*)
Gold-toothed aloe (*Aloe nobilis*)
Heartleaf philodendron (*Philodendron cordatum*)
Hydrangea (*Hydrangea* sp.)
Indian laurel (*Ficus nitida*)
Jerusalem cherry (*Solanum pseudocapsicum*)
Lantana (*Lantana camara*) – berries of some species toxic
Lily of the valley (*Convallaria majalis*)
Majesty (*Philodendron hastatum*)
Marble queen (*Scindapsus aureus*, *Pothos aureus*)
Narcissus (*Narcissus* sp.) – toxic
Needlepoint ivy (*Hedera helix* 'Needlepoint')
Oleander (*Nerium oleander* L.)
Pothos, Devil's ivy (*Scindapsus aureus*)
Red princess (*Philodendron hastatum*)
Rhododendron (*Rhododendron* spp.)
Rhubarb (*Rheum rhaponticum*)
Ripple ivy (*Hedera helix* 'Ripple')
Saddle leaf (*Philodendron selloum*)
Split-leaf philodendron (*Monstera deliciosa*)
Sprengeri fern (*Asparagus densiflorous* 'Sprengeri')
Umbrella plant (*Cyperus alternifolius*)
Weeping fig (*Ficus benjamina*) – possible dermatitis

*Source*: http://www.tortoisetrust.org/articles/houseplants.htm, accessed December 2012, with permission of The Tortoise Trust.

## More specific toxicoses

Veterinarians in the UK are highly recommended to join the Veterinary Poisons Information Service (VPIS). This is a vast database on toxicoses, with a 24-hour emergency line. All species are covered, including chelonia (see http://www.vpisuk. co.uk or telephone 020 7188 0200).

The following table provides some examples of toxicoses in chelonians – it is intended to describe the more common toxins. In keeping with the generalised signs seen in most cases, most cases will require a basic biological support (BBS):

- heat (to recommended preferred optimal temperature zone)
- ultraviolet light

| Type of toxin | Toxin | Examples | Specific signs (if any) | Notes on diagnosis and treatment |
|---|---|---|---|---|
| Plant (see above) | Gastrointestinal irritants (incl. oxalates and alkaloids) | Amaryllis<br>Arrowhead plant<br>Boston ivy<br>Caladium<br>Croton (purgative)<br>Dumbcane<br>Emerald duke<br>Heartleaf philodendron<br>Marble queen<br>Majesty<br>Narcissus<br>Pothos, Devil's ivy<br>Red princess<br>Rhubarb (leaves)<br>Saddle leaf<br>Split-leaf philodendron | Vomiting/diarrhoea<br>Oral mucosal ulceration | In early stages, activated charcoal; later, use sucralfate<br>Orabase gel may be used to cover oral ulcers |
| | Glycosides | Christmas rose<br>Hydrangea<br>Lily of the valley<br>Oleander | Weakness<br>Bradycardia | BBS |
| | Skin irritants | Asparagus fern<br>Chenille plant (also gut irritant)<br>Chrysanthemum<br>Creeping fig<br>Gold-toothed aloe<br>Indian laurel<br>Sprengeri fern | Erythema/ulceration of skin<br>Pruritus | Bathing<br>Dressing of ulcers – see Chapter 33 |
| | Solanine | Bittersweet<br>Jerusalem cherry | Weakness<br>Neurological signs<br>Signs as per gastrointestinal irritants | Treat as gastrointestinal irritants<br>BBS |

| | | |
|---|---|---|
| Rhododendron (contains rhodotoxin and glycosides) | Weakness/paralysis<br>Bradycardia/atrioventricular block<br>Vomiting | In early stages, remove leaves from mouth/stomach if possible by endoscopy<br>In first few hours, give activated charcoal<br>Atropine if severe A-V block (0.02–0.04 mg/kg im q12–24 h)<br>Sucralfate after first day<br>BBS |
| Mushrooms | Lethargy<br>Occasionally, neurological signs (dependent on species ingested) | BBS<br>Diazepam if severe seizures/tremors) - 2.5 mg/kg im/iv as required |
| Iatrogenic | | |
| Ivermectin | Depression<br>Paralysis<br>Coma/death | BBS – recovery may take weeks |
| Vitamin A | Inappetance<br>Full-thickness skin thickening | Seen after injection of high doses of vitamin A; for this reason, vitamin A should always be given orally<br>BBS<br>Dress skin lesions as per Chapter 33 |
| Vitamin D (incl. cholecalciferol rodenticides) | Renal failure secondary to soft tissue mineralisation | Can occur with oral supplements as well as injectable<br>Poor prognosis if mineralisation seen on radiographs<br>Aggressive fluid therapy, BBS and withdrawal of all vitamin D containing supplements |
| Metronidazole | Neurological signs | BBS<br>Diazepam 2.5 mg/kg im/iv |
| Organophosphates and carbamates | Salivation<br>Ataxia<br>Tremors/seizures<br>Coma | More likely to cause problems if given with levamisole/pyrethroids<br>Wash animal after exposure<br>BBS<br>Atropine 0.4 mg/kg im q12–24 h |

(Continued)

| Type of toxin | Toxin | Examples | Specific signs (if any) | Notes on diagnosis and treatment |
|---|---|---|---|---|
| | Pyrethroids | | As organophosphates | Wash thoroughly after exposure as transcutaneous absorption can occur<br>BBS<br>Diazepam 2.5 mg/kg im/iv |
| Heavy metals | Lead | | Neurological signs<br>Haematuria | Blood lead levels diagnostic, though signs and presence of metal in gut on radiographs suggestive<br>BBS<br>Sodium calcium edetate 50 mg/kg im q48h<br>Consider surgical/endoscopic removal of lead source if not expelled normally under chelation |
| | Zinc | | Anorexia/lethargy<br>Enteritis<br>Haematuria<br>Haemolytic anaemia | Signs more chronic than in lead toxicosis<br>Radiography for metal in gut and blood zinc levels useful<br>BBS<br>Sodium calcium edetate 50 mg/kg im q48h<br>Surgical/endoscopic removal of zinc-containing foreign bodies in gut |
| Anticoagulants | Coumarols | | Haemorrhage<br>Petechiation | Can assess/monitor via Buccal Mucosal Bleeding Time or Prothrombin Time; as normals not established, compare with normal animal of same species at same temperature<br>BBS<br>Vitamin K1 2.5 mg/kg im/po q 24h |
| Metaldehyde | Metaldehyde | | Ataxia<br>Incoordination<br>Tremors<br>Seizures<br>Coma | Very poor prognosis<br>BBS<br>Diazepam 2.5 mg/kg im/iv as required; may take days for recovery |

- fluids
- supportive nutrition
- broad-spectrum antibiosis
- regular assessment of hydration and renal function
- oxygen via ventilation if respiratory collapse

## Further reading

Fitzgerald, K. & Newquist, K. (2008) Poisonings in reptiles. *Veterinary Clinics of North America Exotic Animal Practice*, **11**(2), 327–358. This is an excellent reference.

# Index

*Essentials of Tortoise Medicine and Surgery*, First Edition. John Chitty and Aidan Raftery.
© 2013 John Chitty and Aidan Raftery. Published 2013 by John Wiley & Sons, Ltd.

Printed and bound by CPI Group (UK) Ltd, Croydon, CR0 4YY

27/10/2024

14580193-0002